How to help your autistic spectrum child

How to help your autistic spectrum child

Practical ways to make family life run more smoothly

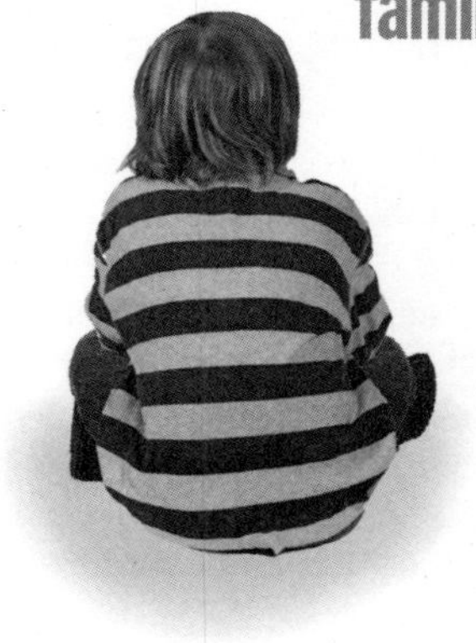

Jackie Brealy and Beverly Davies

Editors: Richard Craze and Roni Jay

Viva Books
New Delhi | Mumbai | Chennai | Kolkata
Bangalore | Hyderabad | Kochi | Guwahati

First Indian Edition 2010

VIVA BOOKS PRIVATE LIMITED

- 4737/23 Ansari Road, Daryaganj, New Delhi 110 002
  E-mail: vivadelhi@vivagroupindia.net, Tel. 42242200
- 76, Service Industries, Shirvane, Sector 1, Nerul, Navi Mumbai 400 706
  E-mail: vivamumbai@vivagroupindia.net, Tel. 27721273, 27721274
- Jamals Fazal Chambers, 26 Greams Road, Chennai 600 006
  E-mail: vivachennai@vivagroupindia.net, Tel. 28290304, 28294241
- B-103, Jindal Towers, 21/1A/3 Darga Road, Kolkata 700 017
  E-mail: vivakolkata@vivagroupindia.net, Tel. 22836381, 22816713
- 7, Sovereign Park Apartments, 56-58, K. R. Road, Basavanagudi, Bangalore 560 004
  E-mail: vivabangalore@vivagroupindia.net, Tel. 26607409, 26607410
- 101-102 Mughal Marc Apartments, 3-4-637 to 641, Narayanguda, Hyderabad 500 029
  E-mail: vivahyderabad@vivagroupindia.net, Tel. 27564481, 27564482
- Beevi Towers, First Floor, SRM Road, Kaloor, Kochi 682 018, Kerala
  E-mail: vivakochi@vivagroupindia.net, Tel: 0484-2403055, 2403056
- 232, GNB Road, Beside UCO Bank, Silpukhuri, Guwahati 781 003
  E-mail: vivaguwahati@vivagroupindia.net, Tel: 0361-2666386

www.vivagroupindia.com

Published by arrangement with

Crimson Publishing,
a division of Crimson Business Ltd
Westminster House, Kew Road
Richmond, Surrey TW9 2ND

ISBN : 978-81-309-1485-5

Published by Vinod Vasishtha for Viva Books Private Limited, 4737/23, Ansari Road, Daryaganj, New Delhi - 110 002.

Printed and bound by Raj Press, R-3, Inderpuri, New Delhi - 110 012.

Contents

The National Autistic Society

The National Autistic Society

Over 535,000 people are affected by autism in the UK alone – around 1 in 110 – and this figure rises to two million when you include parents, carers and siblings whose lives can be turned upside down as a result of living with autism.

The National Autistic Society (NAS) is the UK's leading charity for people with autism and their families and carers. Founded in 1962, the NAS spearheads national and international initiatives and provides a strong voice for all people with autism. The NAS provides a wide range of services helping people with autism and Asperger syndrome to live their lives with as much independence as possible, and supporting their families and carers.

The NAS runs a number of schools, colleges and adult services offering day and residential care for people with autism, as well as a supported employment consultancy called Prospects. The NAS also provides a range of support services for parents and families living with autism, from befriending schemes and social groups, to specific programmes and training schemes for different issues affecting those living with autism.

The NAS' Parent to Parent Helpline is a free, confidential telephone support service offered by volunteer parents to other parents of an adult or child with autism. All our parent volunteers share the determination and experience to offer invaluable help and support to other parents.

For more information about autism and NAS services or to support us, please visit www.autism.org.uk

The National Autistic Society is a registered Charity, number 269425
Head Office: 393 City Road, London, EC1V 1NG, United Kingdom

Tel: +44(0)20 7833 2299, Fax: +44 (0)20 7833 9666, Email: nas@nas.org.uk

Dedication and acknowledgements

JACKIE

I would like to thank my family Keith, Ben, Paul and Zoe for being so supportive, but most of all to Matt for teaching us so much. As Matt says, “Don’t worry, be happy.” And we are.

BEV

Thanks to Neil for being really helpful and kind and for giving me the benefit of his unrivalled pedantry, to Prudy, Henry, Susie and my father, who have all been brilliant while I have been writing this book, also to all the friends who came up with contacts and ideas. I’m sure everyone will understand if I dedicate my half of the book to my mother, who would have been very pleased to see it.

A note to readers

'Autistic Spectrum Disorders' is a title that covers the conditions known as Autism and Asperger's syndrome, generally referred to as ASD within the book.

All the information is given in good faith; it is given for general use and should not be seen as applicable to any individual situation. Anyone seeking advice on health should see their GP or appropriate health professional in the first instance.

Introduction

Getting a diagnosis of Autistic Spectrum Disorder is not the end of the world – but it is the beginning of a journey

A boy is standing at the side of the road. He is screaming and crying and flapping his arms, in a state bordering on complete panic. To an outsider it looks as if he is having a terrible tantrum, but I know there is much more to it than that. His unhappiness is hard to bear. I don't know what to do about it and, of more immediate importance, I don't know how to get him across the road.

My name is Jackie. I live in Devon with my husband and my four children, who range in age from 20 to 10. Because Matt was my third child I knew there was something different about him from day one. He didn't connect, he didn't make eye contact, he didn't walk until he was two and his speech development was very slow. The diagnosis of Asperger's Syndrome was a long time coming. In fact, when we finally knew what was wrong, it was almost a relief to be able to give Matt's problems a name and to feel that we had some idea of what to expect.

Now Matt is 14. He goes to regular school, and a casual observer, seeing him with his friends, would probably think he was a teenager like any other. He is in a band at school, mucks around and gets into a bit of trouble from time to time, just like the rest of the boys. He communicates with other people reasonably well and has pretty good social skills.

I call Matt 'my little Harry Enfield teenager'. The normal teenager and the autistic teenager in him are slightly at loggerheads. He wants to be like everybody else, but he doesn't really know where to draw the line, so he gets into more trouble than the others. He will still sometimes do extreme things – he walked through a bonfire because he wanted to see what it was like (his shoes melted, so I like to think he wouldn't do it again, though of course I cannot rule it out). He still needs routine and likes to know exactly what is happening and when.

It has been a long journey from that terrible day at the side of the road to where we are now, and I want to tell you how we made it.

If you have just had a diagnosis of Autistic Spectrum Disorder (ASD) for your child, don't panic. I just want everyone to know that however bleak the diagnosis can seem, you may well be able to make the sort of progress that we have made with Matt. I don't want to paint a picture that is too rosy, but I have as much pride and joy in Matt as I do in my other children. I think over time, partly because I am now trained in learning support for special needs pupils, partly because I have a habit of observing and analysing behaviour, I have found some good ways of dealing with Matt and his problems, and I would like to share them with you.

It took a long time to get to the bottom of those roadside panics of Matt's, but I got there in the end. At first I didn't understand his anxiety, I thought he was just having a terrible tantrum. I used to pick him up and put him back in his buggy and carry on, even though he was screaming at me. It wasn't until I started to look at just when he was doing it that I realised that there was a pattern. If we were trying to cross the road he would get in a total state and curl up on the pavement, screaming. He would start flapping his arms and would get really panicky. His anxiety went off the scale. I just couldn't say or do anything to control him. He would keep repeating the word 'cars' because he couldn't talk very well at that time. After a while, I understood. He was getting into a state because the cars were coming in too many different directions for him to concentrate on them all.

I needed an idea to help him with crossing the road, so at home we set up his car mat with cars and played at crossing the road using the toy cars so that we could check which side they would come from when you were crossing. Then when we went out we could put into practice which way you would have to look to see the cars coming.

A lot of parents get stuck into the trap of trying to make their child behave in a 'normal' way, rather than trying to understand what the problems are. I always try to be responsive to Matt's problems, just as I was with the cars, and I don't try to make him behave the way my other children behaved. In fact, that would be impossible, because he is so fundamentally different.

Some parents may well think that their child will get over or grow out of these things or that they can simply force him to change, without ever realising that there are reasons for a lot of the strange behaviour or understanding the implacable if bizarre logic behind it. They don't work out how to help their child to cope with whatever is upsetting him.

When we are bringing up our children there are a lot of things that we simply never explain because we assume that they somehow automatically know them, but they may puzzle away at something for ages and worry about it without our realising. We need to see things through children's eyes. Bringing up Matt made me realise that you should never assume they know or understand something. I have to go right back to basics and explain things every time: he can't just accept what I am saying.

With my other children I think I was a run of the mill parent. I can see how I have changed with Matt because he is so different. I often think I should have explained things more to the older two .The experience I have had with Matt has taught me a lot, which I try to relay to other parents through my work, when we talk about the children's worries and try to find a way around them.

Once you know it is an Autistic Spectrum Disorder

- Don't panic. Most situations can be improved.
- Try to look at things through your child's eyes.
- Try to understand your child. If you realise *why* they do things you will begin to see how you can help.
- See what your child does in troublesome situations and

write it down. It is likely that a pattern will start to emerge.

- Be prepared to go over things with them time and time again.
- Love your child for who they are, and help them to be proud of themselves, don't try and change him – but do try to do something about things that cause them problems.
- Take a look at every source of help and advice that comes your way. The more support you can get the better – and that's what this book is for.

Chapter 1

Defining the condition

Autism is a complex developmental disability that affects the way children communicate and relate to the world around them. The spectrum of autism means that children are affected by the condition to different degrees. Over 500,000 people in Britain, according to figures from the National Autistic Society, are somewhere on the spectrum, which ranges from severe autism, through high functioning autism to Asperger's syndrome at the more able end.

If you suspect that your child's behaviour puts them somewhere on the spectrum you may still find that a definitive diagnosis is a long time coming. Autistic difficulties are usually present from birth, though children may appear to develop normally until up to about age two to three before problems become hard to ignore. In the past, many people could not get a diagnosis until their child started school or even later. Now things have improved in this area to the extent that diagnosis – and helpful treatments – can kick in at a much younger age. Although ASDs are not curable, they respond to treatment, especially if this starts as early as possible. If you feel that your child may be affected it is worth pressing for a specialist diagnosis as soon as possible, making your GP your first port of call.

You can see why it can be hard to spot ASDs in very young children. Diagnosis is based on observing behaviour, after all this is a handicap that is social rather than physical. You can only really spot problems with social interaction when a child reaches toddler age, although parents are often sure that there is something amiss from very early on.

Although this is a condition that needs to be diagnosed on a very individual basis, rendering a tick-box list of symptoms unhelpful, there are some factors that will help to point you towards a diagnosis. ASDs affect the way an individual relates to others and communicates with them, disrupting the development of social, communication and cognitive skills. Common factors for both autism and Asperger's syndrome are:

- **difficulty in communicating**
  - problems in understanding language – very literal interpretation with no appreciation of nuance
  - problems in using language – if present, speech patterns are often peculiar
  - problems in recognising or interpreting facial expressions, gestures and tone of voice
- **difficulty in social relationships**
  - can seem aloof and indifferent to people
  - lack of two way social relationships
  - lack of empathy/sympathy – find it hard to understand that others may see things from a different viewpoint
  - sometimes want to establish a relationship but no idea how to do it

- **lack of imagination and creative play**
  - fear of change, preference for sameness
  - restricted interests: limited play

Together, these three areas of difficulty are known as the **triad of impairments**. This triad is often accompanied by a narrow and repetitive pattern of activity that is comforting to the child.

It is important to consider what the triad means to each individual child: the areas of difficulty may not be equally impaired, and the results of impairment may be different at different stages of development, so treatment should always be tailored to the individual.

Children with ASDs find it hard to make sense of what is going on around them. Understanding other people's expressions of emotion can be difficult or impossible for them and it can be very hard to develop friendships. The difficulty people with ASDs have in imagining what someone else may be thinking or feeling is explained by the idea that they lack what is known as a 'theory of mind'. A child with autism may well think that you know everything that they know or think, and it will not occur to them to try to communicate any of it to you.

The need for routine is paramount. When a child has trouble comprehending their environment and no way of predicting what will happen next, then routine is a great source of comfort and safety. Any attempt to vary a routine or pattern may lead to challenging behaviour from the child. However, on the bright side, this dependence on routine and structure can be a positive thing in a classroom context.

Children with Asperger's syndrome are not as withdrawn as classic autists; they often enjoy contact and want to be sociable, though their difficulty in 'reading' social signals from other people can make this hard for them. While people with Asperger's syndrome often speak fluently, they may not take much notice of the reaction of listeners. These children do not necessarily have any of the accompanying learning disabilities associated with autism, and will often enter mainstream school. They can be very good at learning facts and figures, though they do find it hard to think in abstract ways. The idea of the autistic genius is something of a modern myth. In fact ASD IQs go right across the range from genius to severe learning difficulty, and up to 75% of people with ASDs have learning difficulties of some kind.

ASD is:

- a developmental disorder
- associated with unusual response to sensory stimulation
- four times more likely to occur in boys than girls
- found in all social groups

ASD may be:

- genetically linked – you may find other family members with ASD
- accompanied by epilepsy and other disorders such as ADD (attention deficit disorder) and OCD (obsessive compulsive disorder)

- accompanied by particular skills such as music, drawing or maths
- accompanied by moderate or severe learning difficulties

ASD is not:

- caused by parental rejection
- caused by stress, though stress and anxiety may make the symptoms worse

How we got our diagnosis

Because Matt was my third child, I knew from very early on that he was not exactly standard issue. I'm not at all sure that I would have picked things up so quickly if he had been my first. Despite my early worries, it took a long, long time to get a diagnosis, in fact he was nearly eight when we knew for sure.

Apparently autistic children are often late developers, and Matt certainly bore that out. At 18 months he wasn't talking or walking or doing other age-appropriate things. I brought my concerns up with the health visitor but didn't really get anywhere. When Matt was two and a half I went back, and they still said I had to wait until he was a bit older. When he started nursery, still in nappies, they noticed that he was a loner who always played by himself and had no interest in getting to know the other children. The staff found it very hard to get any response from him; he seemed to have no comprehension of what was going on around him.

We had a huge daily battle to get anywhere when Matt was a toddler, he used to flap his hands and get upset in a way that children usually don't, getting very angry about things when they didn't seem to make sense to him. We thought a lot of his temper was because he was frustrated that he couldn't walk yet. When he did start walking he fell over a lot and some of his behaviour was downright disturbing. If we had someone around to visit he would scream all the time. We couldn't sit and talk or chat and have tea, he would just scream. In consequence, we didn't have people around or go out much because it was such a hassle.

Things certainly didn't seem right with Matt, but we didn't know what was wrong. We just thought it was extreme quirky toddler behaviour – we thought his toddler stage was going to last forever. Just to go and do the shopping was a nightmare, getting him dressed was a daily struggle, and the other children were always put on hold. It seemed really wrong.

When I went to the GP my main concern was that Matt never responded to me. I had thought that his hearing might be at the root of it, but that proved to be fine. Then I mentioned his lack of responsiveness, at which stage we were referred to a paediatrician who did the test for epilepsy and sent us on to a child psychologist, who took a history of everything that had happened to Matt from birth onwards.

The tests revealed both epilepsy and Asperger's syndrome. Although I had heard of autism, Asperger's was a completely unknown quantity. When we first got the diagnosis, we were dumbfounded. We didn't know what we needed to do. It took us months to come to terms with it. A disability you can see is much easier to accept than a mental disability. Every time we looked at Matt we couldn't believe what we had been told. He looked so normal and he was such a sweet child in so many ways that I found it very hard to believe that something had gone wrong with his brain.

A lot of parents are reluctant to take their children in to be assessed because they are afraid of that label, and I can understand that. But the label opens up a world for these children to get much more of the help they need, for them to understand why they feel so different from everyone else, and for you, as a parent, to understand them. At the mild end of the spectrum, without a diagnosis it would be possible to go your whole life without knowing why you felt different. If you are older when you find out what is causing your problems, you can start to deal with your condition, and, if you so wish, to break some of the habits that make you look different in society. As an individual, fitting in can help you if you want to be in the group. We all have to modify our behaviour to some extent. As the parent of a child with an ASD, you have to make some of these decisions for them.

I believe that getting the label is better than not knowing, and it has certainly helped with Matt. Some parents give their children all the details of the condition. I didn't choose to do that with Matt. I felt that showing him everything on a list of behaviour would make him think 'well, I have to do this because it is part of my condition and I can't do that because that is part of my condition.' A list like that is both limiting and defining.

However, I am really glad that we got Matt's diagnosis sorted out when he was young. If we hadn't known until later it would have been much harder because there would have been different barriers. It is important to get a diagnosis for practical reasons, too. Diagnosis leads to statementing (discussed in detail in Chapter 13) and, with any luck, to a proper consideration of your child's educational needs. The label may qualify you for Disability Living Allowance or a disabled parking permit, which can certainly make life easier. Really, anything that helps has got to be worth it.

I never want to change Matt: as he once said to me 'Who is different – me or you?' and he has every right to be the person he is.

Recognition of ASD has increased over the last decade since I was looking for answers with Matt. Early diagnosis helps in so many ways. There are lots of things that can be done to help your child, and the sooner you start, the more likely they are to be effective. It can certainly help to get started before behaviour patterns get too entrenched.

If this is your first child you have no point of comparison, so there are things you could easily miss and your worries may only become clear over time. With the late emergence of all the signs, and average gaps between children of two to three years, it is quite likely that by the time you realise that something is seriously amiss with your first child you will either have or be expecting your second.

It is not always easy to get an early diagnosis however sure you are that there is something wrong. We saw five or six people before the diagnosis, and the extent of Matt's problems emerged only gradually. If you notice that your child is a loner, or doesn't make eye contact, or talk, or point at anything when they might be expected to, you might want to look for other things in their behaviour that chime with this diagnosis. There are not many absolute rules, however. Most children with ASD don't want to share information or point out things. Matt would take my hand and lead me to what he wanted me to see, but that is far from typical, he has always been unusually communicative for an ASD child. If you are worried, make a list of your concerns and take them to your GP.

A word about CHAT

CHAT stands for Checklist of Autism in Toddlers and is a screening tool developed at Cambridge University's Autism Research Centre. It consists of a series of simple, but defining questions for parents and GP, such as whether the child points at things to show interest in them, enjoys pretend play or takes an interest in other children. The researchers suggest that it should be included in the GP's 18 month check of all toddlers. This does not happen at present but, if you have concerns, you could ask your GP to do the test [details can be found on the National Autistic Society website **www.autism.org.uk** or the PEACH (Parents for the early intervention of autism in children) website **www.peach.org.uk**.] With an eye to the effectiveness of early intervention, it is worth pressing for a diagnosis if you have worries, and, while not in itself a diagnosis, this is a substantial first step.

What if you have trouble getting a diagnosis?

It can be dreadful for parents who know something is wrong, suspect it is ASD and cannot convince health professionals.

This can be a very isolating experience and, alas, is not uncommon. If you are having trouble getting a diagnosis:

- Find out the way through the maze from support groups (The National Autistic Society could be your first port of call) and fellow parents.
- A written diagnosis, where a health professional writes that your child has an autistic spectrum disorder, is essential if you and your child are to get the help and support you need.
- Try to work with the professional and avoid conflict, even if you disagree. Give a clear summary of your child's problems. Some professionals are against 'labelling' children, but the 'label' given by a clear diagnosis is the only way to get the help they need.
- Make sure you feel happy that you have a complete diagnosis. Remember that ASD goes right across the spectrum of intelligence – so a child's intelligence levels have nothing to do with whether or not they are in the ASD spectrum. Many other disorders such as OCD, ADD or challenging behaviour can be a part of the ASD, so if you feel you have not received a complete diagnosis, keep going.
- Accept that it can take time – a lot of time – to get the clear diagnosis you need. You have to trust your instincts as a parent – you know your child better than anyone.
- The Elizabeth Newson Centre in Nottingham helps parents of children with developmental communication disorders to obtain a specialist diagnostic assessment of their child as

early as possible. The centre is a charity and parents can make a direct referral, although for funding purposes it is probably best to be referred by your GP or paediatrician. (01623 490879) **www.sutherlandhouse.org.uk.**

Dealing with the Triad

There is only so much you can do here, you are dealing with a person and you can't make parts of their personality go away, but there are things you can try that may help in almost every area.

- **Difficulty understanding language** – use one of the specially developed communication systems (PECS for straightforward communication, Makaton where things are more severe – details in chapter 2), also audiotapes, and, if your child likes TV, use videos to help you or even make your own. You can use a camcorder to make a short film on aspects of daily life, like dressing, or eating at the table, introducing members of the family over and over again until the child starts to recognise them.
- **Difficulty showing or understanding emotions** – when they smile say 'that's a lovely happy face', when they cry say 'you are so sad' underlining the emotion they were feeling. Get them to draw someone's happy face, so they associate the feeling with a person.
- **Difficulty with social interaction** – if they are cut off encourage them to socialise. This would not work for children who are really isolated in their autism. With such children I would see if I could find something they liked so that I could get a

connection going. Sit nearby, playing with something they might find interesting, and let them come to you.

- **Difficulty with two way social relationships** – ask them for more information, and more and more. In the end it will have to become a dialogue. For turn taking play games with a couple of children and say 'Jackie's go', 'Michael's go' 'soon your go, Fred, wait for your turn' and repeat endlessly until, with luck, the penny drops.
- **Lack of empathy** – they won't understand how their words can make people feel. Say similar things back to them: 'you look spotty', 'why is your hair a mess?' and try to get them to see that it is not very nice to be on the receiving end of such comments. Get a 'feelings' book that contains pictures of people showing various different emotions in different situations.
- **No idea how to form friendships** – teach them to go up to someone and say 'can I play?' If they start doing this at a young age they will not be so self-conscious.
- **Lack of imagination** – show a picture then prod them to think about it with questions such as 'do you think the child in the picture is happy or sad?' so you are getting them to use some imagination and make up a story.
- **Fear of change** – change is a part of life and I think ASD children have to learn to accept it. Don't entirely protect them from it, but be supportive if it causes problems, and put strategies in place to make it easier to cope with.
- **Restricted interests / limited play** – ASD children are likely to

have their obsessions, and not want to look beyond them for play. Offer them something extra to play with: expand one game with extra components.

- **Need for routine and repetition** – if this is not causing a family problem it is probably best to go along with your child's rituals as much as possible. For help when it does become a problem, see Chapter 8.

Chapter 2

The importance of starting early

In the bad old days, when it was unusual to get a diagnosis of autism at a young age, lots of opportunities for helping and understanding ASD children were lost. Even now, although diagnosis may come by around age two, this is not always the case.

Early intervention, however, is very much to be hoped for: it can reduce the build-up of behavioural problems and stop some habits from becoming too entrenched. As the difficulties of the triad relate to every aspect of a child's life, so across-the-board parental involvement is extra important. Some things just evolve naturally at home, and there are some very helpful programmes that parents can get involved in.

Learning with pictures

When Matt was small I started using pictures that were relevant to him to help. I didn't know it then, but this is a standard treatment. At the time it was just a system I evolved myself because I had to find a way for Matt to understand me more quickly as my two older children needed me too. He responded to the pictures, which really helped. Then he started mimicking me and now his verbal skill is fantastic but when he is cross he still reverts to pictures. I keep little round disc pictures of happy, sad, angry and worried faces on the fridge for him, to help him express emotions when he can't find the words. If he puts up the angry face picture then he can have time out in his bedroom and he is grateful then that I knew what he needed, that he couldn't quite express for himself.

Initially, to help him with getting dressed, I used photographs of his actual clothes stuck onto the drawers they were in, so that he could see at a glance where they were. I started that when he was two and kept it going until he was about eight, when he finally clicked that things were always in the same drawer. The dressing routine involved me telling him the things to put on in order as I went to and fro past his room in the morning, and gradually, over time, he got his own routine going.

Difficulty with social communication is a key factor in ASD and one way of addressing it is through the use of picture symbols. Children with ASD tend to be visual learners, so pictures can help them make sense of the world. Photographs, line drawings, objects and written words can be helpful ways to accompany and augment speech but, as in so many areas, ASD makes communication more complicated. Children with ASD may find a line drawing less confusing than a photo. They may register details more strongly than the whole thing, and so can be confused if a photo used does not correspond exactly with the object that it symbolises. For instance, they will see that a line drawing of 'crisps' relates to all crisps, where they can't see that a picture of a particular brand has anything at all in common with any other crisps.

PECS (The Picture Exchange Communication System)

PECS was developed to help young children with autism to learn how to initiate requests and communicate what they need. They have to learn how communication works, which is hard for them. The basic understanding that another person may not know what you want until you tell them is missing in their make-up, so they do not intrinsically understand the need to communicate. For example, an ASD boy who is thirsty assumes his mother knows that he wants a drink. If, knowing he is thirsty, she hasn't produced a drink, there is no point in asking her for one. Children can learn how communication works if they are taught to exchange a symbol for something they want. PECS has proved to be very effective, it is easy to use and involves no expensive equipment, testing or training, though professionals and parents can take training courses.

The earlier the children start PECS the better. You will communicate more quickly with them and will have less anxiety to deal with as, from an early age, children who have mastered it will be used to being able to tell you what they want.

First associate the picture symbol with the actual thing it represents, by attaching a paper symbol to the object (eg 'biscuit'). When the child has started to associate the symbol with the real thing, then an identical symbol a little away from the actual thing lets the parent or carer show the symbol while telling the child what to get. Symbols should be used first with things that motivate the child, such as 'biscuit', or 'drink', and the rate at which they can be introduced varies from child to child.

By establishing the individual child's likes among food and toys he is taught in a step-by-step process to exchange a symbol for the item he wants. There are six carefully structured stages of PECS.

1 the child learns the picture exchange.

2 the child actively finds someone to give a symbol to as a request.

3 the child discriminates between several symbols.

4 the child uses a portable communication book containing picture symbols.

5 the child constructs simple sentences, both requests and comments.

6 the child gradually achieves independence from the helper's prompts and learns that communication is a two-way process which gets the desired results.

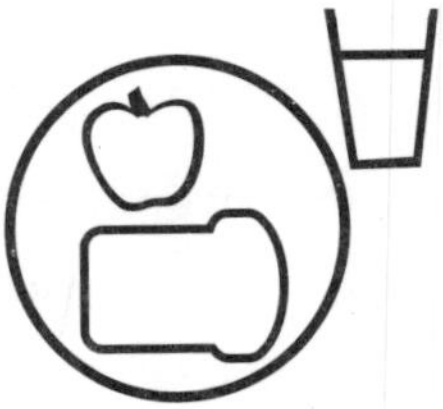

lunchtime

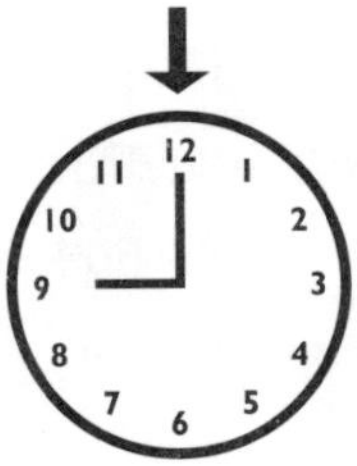

now

PECS often helps in the development of spoken words and encourages interaction, and possibly eye contact, as the children have to find someone to give the symbol to. Children learn to communicate using PECS because they are motivated to get something they want. With severely autistic children who cannot communicate verbally, all they use is their PECS book. For my ASD students I get a small diary and put in a sheet to which I attach all the pictures that describe their day at school. If the children want to communicate something they learn to use the PECS picture of a drink if they want a drink, and so on, and if they want to tell you something they show you in the book. The picture symbols can help make their environment predictable and organised, which helps them keep calm.

Parents should persevere for ages with PECS. It takes the children a long time to realise what the cards are for, so you have to plug away for as much as a year, but then you have opened up a channel of communication that is invaluable. Some autistic children can have a photo of Mummy and not recognise that it is Mummy, so you have to make sure that the pictures they have do mean something to them.

PECS further information from Pyramid Educational Consultants UK Ltd, Pavilion House, 6/7 Old Steine, Brighton BN1 1EJ (01273 609555) **www.pecs.org.uk** For a fee they can send a consultant for a home visit to get you started.

Choices and changes

Picture symbols can be very useful when introducing the idea of choices, such as different foods or play activities. Here the benefit can be encouraging the children to think about trying an available activity that they may enjoy, rather than sticking to one repetitive activity or remaining passive.

Another useful tool is a 'changes' card, which shows them that what they were expecting to do has changed. This card becomes very familiar, which helps them to be less anxious about changes in their daily schedule that would otherwise make them very concerned; it works right across the spectrum, even quite severely autistic children come to recognise it.

Expressing anxiety

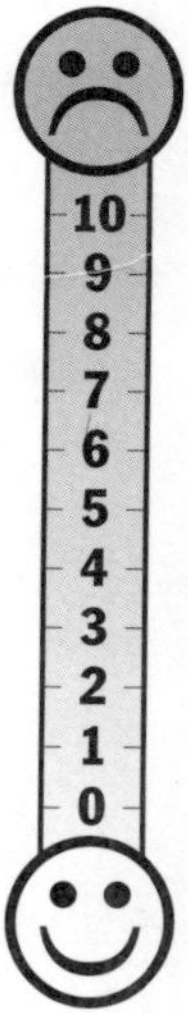

Again, when feelings boil over, a visual method is often the best way to express it. Have a big drawing of a thermometer somewhere in the house with zero at the bottom and numbers going up to ten at the top. Children can point out how angry they are feeling – and sometimes this is much better than putting it into words. When they show you that their anger is starting to build up you can do something about it straight away.

Applied Behavioural Analysis – the Lovaas Programme

This form of behavioural therapy is based on more than 30 years of clinical experience and research carried out by Dr O. Ivar Lovaas in the USA and has been available for some 15 years in this country. It is ideally an early intervention programme for children with ASD, and operates as an intensive home-based regime, targeting the learning of skills broken down into small, achievable steps, taught in a very structured way with a lot of praise and reinforcement. It focuses on one to one teaching undertaken by sets of tutors, and takes one thing at a time, concentrating on and repeating it until the child is seen to have truly learned it. It is very individual; learning blocks as simple as pointing to something or clapping hands are chosen for each child, and every small success is rewarded.

Anne Smith is an ABA therapist and has seen the benefits the programme can bring to parents as well as children. 'The programme is good for parents, not least because every day when they wake up it gives them targets. In a situation where maybe a child seems isolated from the family all the time life can seem terrifyingly without structure. This gives a structure. If they have a goal – to teach the child to clap his hands or put one brick on top of another – at least for part of the day they have something to work on which is for the benefit of their child. The programme can be quite a challenge for parents. The hours are long – as much as 40 hours a week – and the house is full of people all the time.

'I get so much enjoyment from the work. I love the children and the reward, when you get them to make a pile of bricks or whatever, is enormous. Finding the things to do for some of them is very, very hard, because they don't like toys or playing, but there is always something; whether they like being tickled, thrown in the air or watching twinkling lights. Whatever it is you can find it by watching them and then slowly, when they are comfortable with you, you can get them to do some little thing, whether it is take a crisp or clap their hands and you can build up from there. Some of them never get beyond the early stages. I had one little boy who after three years still couldn't say anything, though he could do every puzzle under the sun, was toilet trained and could go to the shops with his mother. There are so many ways of measuring success.

'There is no such thing as a 'cure', what we hope we are doing is helping to make things easier. I feel very privileged that I have had the opportunity to be involved and to see these children for the wonderful kids they are. They all have something special. There is this terrible myth of these sad children and nearly all the ones I have worked with have had a fantastic sense of humour.'

Alexander Lubbock did the Lovaas programme when he was tiny, and his father feels that it gave him a fantastic kick start. 'It is tremendously intense, we had five therapists and 40 hours a week of one to one for him. Each therapist does exactly the same thing with exactly the same words until the child gets it right five times out of five with each therapist, whatever the task is, and then they move on to the next thing. It just cuts through the glass ceiling.'

Alexander is now in school, which is the aim of most parents who do the home programme. There are a few opportunities to pursue ABA in schools that have been set up by parents, so that, at the age of five, children can go there and continue what they have learned at home.

Information from Peach, (01344 882248) **www.peach.org.uk**. This is a parent-led charity which promotes early behavioural intervention for young children with autism using ABA. The service can be funded by your Local Education Authority in some cases, but parents often have to fund the programme themselves.

The EarlyBird Programme

The EarlyBird Programme run by the National Autistic Society lasts three months and consists of group training sessions for parents, combined with individual home visits where video feedback helps parents apply what they learn while working with their child. It supports parents at what can be a difficult time after diagnosis and before school placement and helps them to understand and deal with their child's autism in a way that will help his behaviour and social communication as well as giving invaluable contact with others in the same boat. 'The support of going for ten weeks and having a speech and language therapist, educational psychologist and someone within our borough who knew where to access help and support groups and so on was invaluable,' says Lesley Burton, who found the support on offer a great feature of the course, which she took at a vulnerable time just after her son's diagnosis of autism.

EarlyBird Centre, 3 Victoria Crescent West, Barnsley, S. Yorks S75 2AE (01226 779218 details on **www.autism.org.uk**

Home-Start

This is a brilliant scheme where a helper will befriend you and give you support. A volunteer from the organisation, who is a parent who has been specially trained for the work, comes to your house and helps you to cope with your child so you don't feel so alone. I had one – she would come around, make me a coffee, make sure I got a break while she would play with all the children, not just Matt. It was just what I needed. Find out more through your social worker or at **www.home-start.org.uk**.

Portage

This is a pre-school home visiting service in which a portage worker will regularly visit you to show you how to do interactive play and learning activities with your special needs child and advise on some aspects of child care. Then you practise the activities, which are all based on play, between visits, and report on your child's progress. You can get information on the service through your health visitor or from the National Portage Association (**www.portage.org.uk**). Portage teachers generally have great experience with ASD children and can give you masses of useful advice and support. I think you and your child will both benefit if you start on this as early as possible, before the child gets set in ways and habits. One of the best things about it is the emphasis on what parents can do for their children with appropriate encouragement.

Hanen

Hanen Programmes (run by specially trained Speech and Language Therapists) are based on a US system that aims to teach parents and other care givers ways to promote children's language development during everyday activities. Find out more at **www.hanen.org** .

Makaton

The Makaton Vocabulary is a language programme in which the most frequently used words are matched to British sign language signs and clear picture symbols, all combined to promote communication and encourage language development in children with communication difficulties. At first signs are used and then gradually, if things go according to plan, the signs are dropped and speech takes over. Training programmes in this straightforward system are available for subscribing parents (ask your social worker about help towards the course) and follow-up support is available from a network of trained professionals. Details on **www.makaton.org** (01276 61390). I did one of the courses, and found it a great help, especially for parents whose child doesn't have much communication. Don't be nervous about doing this course. Sitting in a classroom singing a nursery rhyme and signing it at the same time is really great. All the children seem to join in, even those who are severely autistic – this is inclusion in action.

Learning through play

It is always worth making the time to play with your ASD child, they will learn such a lot from it. With severely autistic children you already know they don't want physical contact. Matt's case is milder, but when he was young he would offer me just a part of him to hug – he would never hurl himself into my arms like a normal toddler. Now he is quite cuddly, we have taught him to be, partly through the example of his big brothers, partly through play.

I have endlessly played games where I have said things like 'I am going to cuddle dolly and it will make him feel better because dolly is feeling sad, now.' This helped Matt to learn emotions that he didn't really feel for himself. For instance, one day when I cut myself in the kitchen he said 'you must need a cuddle because you have hurt yourself', but he would not have felt that for himself. Now he comes and gives spontaneous hugs and says 'I love you'. When he was younger it was clearly something learned that he felt was the right thing to say or do, but now he means it. Some ASD children really don't understand the concept of love, they have to learn it. Others may not be able to say it but when you look at them their eyes show liking or love even if they can't express it.

Parents can help them discover feelings and imagination and emotions through play. 'The dolly is sad'; 'the dolly is happy'; 'I love the dolly'. Keep going with all this for years and it pays off: in the end it may become what they mean, not what they have learned. I think this could work with quite severely autistic children too. They do tend to shut themselves away, but you can, while remaining respectful of their condition, try to get through to them with play. You have to allow that they can't always cope with contact and will always need time out from it, but if you can touch them for a few minutes a day you achieve something.

One child I worked with wouldn't make eye contact at all, she would always look down at my feet, so I made some cut-out paper eyes and stuck them on my feet. She looked at the eyes there for a while, and then I slowly moved them up my body over a period of six months or so until they ended up on my forehead, then I took them away and she looked at my real eyes. Then I knew that I had made contact and we made a game where I would say 'look at my eyes' and we would play eye-rolling type games and it took away her fear of eye contact.

Toy story

Set up by Lesley Burton, who was amazed that she couldn't find a shop or mail order catalogue selling the kind of toys she wanted for her autistic son, Eddie, the SenseToys website (**www.sensetoys.com**) features colourful, fun toys and lots of inspiring ideas for how to play with them with your special needs child. Proving that the best toys can often be the least expensive, the brightly coloured Squirmy Wormy Ball, costing just £2.10, is stretchy, easy to catch and can be used to impart the mysteries of turn taking, sharing, hide and seek and lots more besides. Beautiful colourful wooden threading fruits encourage counting, sorting and hand-eye co-ordination.

The toys are carefully chosen to appeal to children with special educational needs – there are lots of play tips and explanations of why each toy meets specific needs. It is truly a family business – each month Eddie's Choice, a favourite toy, is offered at a special price. Lesley says 'I set up the website because I wanted to let people know what was out there. It is a compilation of all that I have learned and been told about from speech and language therapists, child psychologists, special needs teachers, Montessori teachers and other professionals that we have worked with. It is all very well having special toys but if you don't know what to do with them or how to engage your child it is not much use. It is not the toy, it is what you do with it that gives it value for an autistic child. The website is full of play ideas that people seem to find very helpful. It encourages parents to know they are not the only ones whose child is throwing things over his head and not seeming interested in anything. There are a lot of really great ideas in a book called *Playing, laughing and learning with children on the autism spectrum* by Julia Moor, which I sell on the website along with various other helpful books.'

Chapter 3

All about Matt

How it feels to be autistic by Matthew Keith Brealy

'I don't know how you feel so how can I say how I feel, I feel normal thank you.'

I'm going to describe Matt and all his funny ways. I thought he should have one chapter that was just about him, and you will be able to see if you recognise anything similar in your own child. Children with ASD all have their own distinct personalities, yet at the same time there are many characteristics that they seem to have in common.

Well, where do I start: he is my son and I love him, he is tall with brown hair and brown eyes, he likes music, cars and enjoying life to the max. Matt does not like school very much and, like most teenagers, can't wait to leave. Matt likes things his way and to know exactly when/ where/ how things are going to happen. He forgets to finish things you give him to do, like chores around the house or washing himself using soap.

Matt's temper is hot and cold, one minute he is happy, the next he is destroying his room; anything can trigger him off.

Matt likes to socialise with his mates as much as possible, which is very nice to see. He is a very caring boy to his family and would do anything to help when he knows you really need him. Matt will say exactly what is on his mind to anyone. If you ask him 'do you like my dress?' make sure you really want the answer that he will give you!

At home by Matthew Keith Brealy

'Well I have one sister and two brothers so my Mum finds it hard so would I if I was in her position. I have my own room because I used to keep my older brothers awake so now I have been put in my new room sometimes my Mum and Dad find it hard to look after me because they have to keep repeating things what I do not understand and maybe when I have fits it must be scary to watch it happen. Well we all manage and they help me a lot and so do my older brothers and my little sister.'

ASD children's senses are not the same as ours. When Matt was younger every day was a new day for all the impressions that he got and each everyday thing that he saw was a new thing. He was always smelling and tasting things in the house and garden or at the shops, as a way of getting to know them. Now he will say something like 'you've changed the colour of the washing up liquid' rather than having to taste it. That is after many years of telling him not to do it. His sense of taste is quite different – he finds some sweet things bitter and he can't stand to eat anything slimy.

Matt smells things very quickly – people or things. A lot of his judgements on people are based on smell, touch or other senses. His way of identifying things has to be very physical. He has to know what everything he encounters smells and tastes like. Even clothes. If you come into the house he will know if you smell different to normal. For instance, if something has been at my sister's house and then it comes back to me Matt will know that it has been there. So some of his senses are very, very sharp compared to what might be considered the norm.

Really, all his senses are a bit different. His hearing was so sensitive when he was small that he couldn't stand the noise of fireworks, or anything like that, and he still hates loud noises to this day. He could never bear the touch of a hat. When he was a baby he would bite scream and scratch when I put his hat on, and of course with no idea of the problem, I would keep putting it back on. Now he will put a hat on himself but he still hates anybody touching his head. Matt's sight and visual perception are affected. The way he looks at things is different. He sometimes feels as if he sees ceilings or walls closing in on him.

Matt's pain threshold is different from ours so he will do things like hurt his sister to see why she cries. When he was small he put his hand on the heater and held on to it until he had burned his hand so badly it was totally blistered. He doesn't have the wiring to make him feel pain like we do so he is puzzled and asks things like 'why do you cry when you hit your head?'

Pain by Matthew Keith Brealy

'The one good thing about having autism is I don't feel pain like you. I had my finger shut in a door and had to have lots of needles put in my fingernail

but it did not hurt. I also had a nail go through my finger everyone was worrying about it but I got it out with Dad's pliers. It was ok, that made me laugh because everyone else had worried faces.'

Matt has always liked music. With music you play the notes and it comes out how you are playing them. He likes the structure. He was never allowed to learn piano at primary school because he was so far behind academically, but when he did start piano lessons it was clear that he had a natural talent. He has picked up the guitar for himself, and he has even learned to play the drums. He loves listening to music and he can analyse it and tell me all about the structure, which at first amazed me because we are not really a musical family.

How the others see Matt

Ben, (21): 'At the end of the day he is my brother. I would look after him and make sure he is ok. He is harder to control than a normal brother, you have to tell him about 70 times not 20 to do something. When he was younger it was hard as he was in the same bedroom and all night he was shouting or doing something and this was hard to cope with.'

Paul, (18): 'He was hard to deal with when he was small. I felt Mum was with him more than me, but I know now that she had to be with him. It was a nightmare when we shared a bedroom. Now I find he tries to copy me, he mimics me when out or at home. I love him to bits but sometimes I have to stop and look at him and count to ten as I know it is not his fault that he is a pain or doing something wrong. I will always be there for him no matter what he does, he's my bro.'

Zoe, (10): 'I find it hard to do things with him as he gets frustrated, he scares me by jumping out of the cupboard which I hate. I will tell him what to do when he gets older to help him as he needs it. When he has fits I get scared but I have to get used to it and learn what to do when this happens. When I was younger and needed Mum's help and Matt needed her too I used to say help Matt first.'

Keith (Matt's Dad): 'At first I blamed myself for Matt's problems, sometimes seeing myself in the things that he does, but over time and with Jackie's determination we have realised that Matt will not succeed in life skills unless we help him. I now look back over the years with a smile because of all the things that Matt has done: kept me awake at night with his night terrors, insisting that I put him to bed and make sure there are no spiders in the room and that his curtains are right, teasing me constantly and keeping me on my toes, as he often says. Matt has become a loving, caring teenager and I am proud of his determination to do things. Being a teenager is a difficult time for any child and Matt is having some problems dealing with this time in his life but he knows that he can turn to me if he needs help or fatherly advice. I love him to bits, after all he is my son!'

My family by Matthew Keith Brealy

'I love Ben as a brother I will help him if he needs me, I like it when he helps me out when I am in trouble, I can phone him and he will come and help me.

I understand Paul more than anyone he knows a lot more than other people, he has been there and done it. I love him a lot. Paul will always help me out, even if he has important things to do, he always puts family first. Paul has taught me to stick up for myself, if I got beaten up he would come and sort it out.

Zoe has helped me out with lots of things like reading, homework and I will always look after her. She makes me laugh when I am upset and I love her.

Mum is very helpful and has kept me in school throughout the years she has taught me a lot of things to do and what not to do. She tries her best to treat

me like any other kid (like my brothers) what I am glad of. Mum lets me do things so I have had a go at anything, even things that scare me.

Dad helps me out a lot he treats me like a son but talks to me like a best mate, he has taught me to be careful and he lets me do most things that anyone else can do. He has made me more aware of things and has given me a taste of the real world. We have a good laugh together.'

Chapter 4

How ASD affects the family – questions and answers

Getting a diagnosis for your child is only the beginning. This is something that will have repercussions throughout the family, and how your extended family responds may have an impact on how you feel about them. No two families are alike, but from my own experience, and the things I have been asked in my work with other families, I find that some questions crop up over and over again, so I'll tell you about the things that happened to us, what I think we got right, and even some of the things that went a bit wrong.

I have learned a lot from the experience of bringing up Matt, both from the point of view of a parent trying to find the best way through the maze and because the challenges have led me back into education myself. I have done a number of courses and now teach special needs children as a Learning Support Assistant.

When Matt was born my older sons, Ben and Paul, were six and three respectively and I had been with my husband Keith for 18 months. We had settled happily into being a family unit, I used to love those days when we would pack up a picnic or go to the beach just without thinking about it. If we had people round it didn't matter. In retrospect, life was really easy in those days. The boys were so excited about having a new brother, and when Matt was born they adored him. We sometimes feel that we have been tested to the max as a family since then, but here we all are, still together, still happy.

When is the best time to tell your child they are autistic?

I don't think Matt knew he was different when he was small, it was only as he was growing up that he would ask questions like 'why am I different?'

I didn't want Matt to have excuses in his mind for not doing things, so I told him about aspects of his condition as he needed to know them. It is too easy for these children to blame the ASD for everything. It becomes a way of not dealing with things. On the other hand, when they are older it can be quite a relief to understand their condition better and to discover 'oh, that's why I do this.'

The best advice on when to raise the subject comes straight from the horse's mouth. Luke Jackson is a teenager with Asperger's who says, in his book *Freaks, Geeks and Asperger Syndrome* 'My first reaction was relief…If anyone is wondering when to tell their child that they have AS, then, in my humble opinion, the answer is right now!'

- Observe your child and see if the understanding is there before you talk to him about it; ask him if he knows what autism is.
- Try to give him a positive image of himself. Use family photos and videos in which he features and talk about

events he has taken part in so that he can see the role he plays in activities.

How do you explain to a child what autism is?

I did it in stages with Matt. I started by explaining, 'you think differently to other people, so you have to be a bit more patient with them and they have to be a bit more patient with you.' Then, when he was getting into arguments with people because he didn't understand what they were saying, I told him, 'they don't understand why you feel this way because you think differently to them.'

- Give a basic medical explanation of the condition, but keep it simple. Some books can help, but see what you think for your individual child, keep the explanation child-friendly, and don't go into the limitations ASD can impose.

What did Matt make of it?

The christmas Matt was nine he wrote a letter to Santa, he gave me the letter and asked me when I saw Santa could I ask him to keep his stocking and let him be normal for one day so he could see and feel like us. I kept the letter because it was so heartbreaking to realise how much he wanted to understand people and how different from everyone else he felt.

That letter displays a kind of sensitivity that you wouldn't necessarily associate with the condition. I had to explain that Santa couldn't answer individual wishes like that, but I said I would try to help Matt understand. After that, when anything cropped up I would say, 'if that happened it would make me

Hi Santa

I would Like to See you
Some of my Friends say that your not true. I bleve in you are you my best Friend. I think that your the kindess person ever. I have a promlem its horble its Like everone diffend than me. I would Like to Be you.

can I ask some ~~qeion~~ quaion

1. want is it like going arael the word.

2. How old are you.

good bye

From matt

and I tried to be good
you are a very nia man

really happy, or really upset or it would hurt me,' so that he could get some idea of the consequences of actions, and it showed him the difference between how he felt and how I felt in a particular situation.

- Help your child to understand other people's emotions. Collect up pictures from magazines and newspapers of people showing emotions such as anger, excitement and surprise and talk about them.

Does an older child need to know more?

After Matt wrote his letter to Santa, I felt I needed to explain more about his condition. By the time he went to secondary school, he knew it had a name. I explained what it meant and some of the technical aspects of the condition. I told him about some of the famous people who were autistic and other things that would help him to have a more positive impression. Then luckily there was something on television about a mathematical genius who had Asperger's. He watched it and accepted all that.

I didn't tell him the things that he would not be able to do. I told him that there was probably no point in his reading about it, as each person with autism is different and while he might have some of the things they wrote about he might not have any of them. If he had wanted to know more I would have highlighted the aspects that might apply to him and not have shown him any more than that. In fact, he didn't want to see anything. He knew that he would be able to do things like preparing his meals and having a job – we always emphasised the positive. As he has got older Matt has become more analytical of the differences between him and us.

What to tell ASD children – and when

- Emphasise the positive in terms of what they *can* do.
- Tell them about famous people who have had the same condition: there is speculation that such well-known figures from the past as Albert Einstein, Isaac Newton and even Andy Warhol may have displayed behavioural patterns linked to ASD.
- Each child is different but for almost all of them it will be a

relief to know that there is a reason why they feel the way they do.

- You don't have to tell them everything at once. You will know best how much they can take in at any given time, and how much it is helpful for them to know about the condition.
- It may help to explain how you feel in particular situations and how it is different to how they feel.

As the mother of an academically gifted Asperger's sufferer, Finni Golden felt the same as I did when it came to telling her son, Jamie, about his condition. 'Knowing that Jamie has Asperger's has made a huge difference to both of us; the worry that he had when he couldn't understand why he was different and why he found things so difficult was far worse. Once you know that you have a problem you can address it and it is part of knowing who you are. He suffers badly with Obsessive Compulsive disorder as well, but I never made him think that he was ill; I just explained that everyone has tidiness parameters and all these other things but there are always going to be people who are off the scale and that he is a little bit off the scale, and then I told him about some scientific research, which helps to explain how he is about things. They did an experiment where they showed people with Asperger's syndrome flash cards of an object and then a face. In a 'normal' brain you analyse the face and expressions in a different area of your brain to a table or chair, whereas with someone with Asperger's it all goes into the same place. This may be why they can't read facial expressions and also why they are not considerate of other people's feelings. My son is enormously good company and he is very funny so there is absolute delight alongside all the horrendous things.'

When do you tell siblings and how can you expect them to react?

My advice to parents would be to explain as soon as you can. Start by keeping it simple. Depending on their ages, you could just say something like 'your brother is different and we can all help him in different ways.' As the siblings get older you can explain more. Younger siblings have to get used to it all bit by bit. You need to explain that lots of things that they do without thinking – like making eye contact, taking turns and understanding what other people are thinking and feeling – are very hard for their brother or sister with an ASD.

Mine knew quite early on – before Matt did really – and our youngest child, Zoe, who is five years younger than Matt, knew there was something different about her brother from a very early age. She was quite a laid back baby and if she heard Matt scream she would automatically be quiet. I could deal with him and then go back to her, even if I had been in the middle of feeding her, which is not normal, but was just what I needed. I thought she was sent from heaven. When she was about three if Matt was in a state she would say 'Mummy go to Matt first' because she knew I had to sort him out, and she still has a lot of patience with him to this day.

The older two found it very hard sometimes when they were younger. Matt used to upset them with things like tearing up their homework and keeping them awake at night. Just try telling your teacher that your brother has destroyed your homework. It may be a novel twist on 'the dog ate it' but it does not go down any better. He would take something from one brother and put it in the other one's bag because he found it fascinating to see them getting angry. When they were all sharing a room he would swap their teddy bears around when they were asleep. It was all quite ingenious, but he really just wanted to see what would happen. He would let the tyres down on their bikes just to see if it would irritate them. Children are very territorial with their things – Matt would sit back and just find it funny. Of course all that was hard for young boys to cope with, but as they have got older they cope really well.

How do you keep the family balance when the siblings inevitably don't get enough attention?

We didn't go out as a family nearly so much when Matt's behaviour started to be challenging. We didn't go on camping holidays with the children until he was older as we knew he couldn't cope with it, which meant that the others missed out. They always had to wait. I think Matt's siblings missed out on normal family social life. It took me a long time to get back into any kind of normal pattern.

The important thing is, we are a family and we are all in it together. Our oldest son has never resented it; the next one down needed more time than I had to give him and I think he did resent that. He is a very sensitive child and he needed me a lot more. He used to get cross with me and say 'you spend all your time with Matt'. I have always regretted it, and you can never put that time back. Now that he is older he knows that he can pick times when I am there for him. He has had to learn how to choose those times.

It was always 'can you do that for yourself, I've just got to go and see to Matt.' The boys used to say ' it's Matt, Matt all the time.' I would suddenly ask 'where is he?' and he would be upstairs drinking the bleach. I could lock it away but he was so smart at finding keys, climbing things, anything. I thought it had to stop because the other children were not having the family life they should be having. That was when the respite care came in, and it was so important to us that I am going to discuss it at length in Chapter 5.

How much can your other children be expected to contribute to the care of a sibling with problems?

Growing up with a brother with special needs has made my children more aware of people around them. It has given them more empathy towards other people. If your children have never been in contact with it, they don't know how to react to disability of any kind and I think that puts them at a disadvantage.

However, we are still in a battle where Matt always needs to come first. We are always thinking about where he is, what he is doing, how he is behaving, and that never ends. Matt doesn't think before things happen and he has always been that way. Even now the older ones will go out and look for him if he has gone off somewhere, just to be on the safe side.

Siblings may find that, as in our family, the ASD child will connect most strongly with one of them. Matt's closest relationship is with my second son, Paul, who is nearest to him in age. Matt has a real admiration for him. When Matt went to his brothers' school Paul was very protective of him, which Matt loved. Paul is quite streetwise so no-one messes with him. If Matt was ever bullied, as soon as the perpetrators realised that Paul was his brother, they left Matt alone. Paul also helps him sort right from wrong. I do ask Paul to chat with Matt if I am not getting through to him.

Are sibling support groups helpful?

I found a group for the siblings of autism or Asperger's children, and the older boys went together. All the children could freely ask the doctor what they wanted to know so the boys found out some of the reasons why Matt did the things he did, which made them feel less alone. Afterwards, when they had talked to other children who were in the same boat as they were, they understood Matt much better, asked me lots of questions about his condition and treatment, and had more patience with him. It might be better for children who are shy of groups to talk to a child psychologist on an individual basis – at any rate, siblings do need some kind of help, you have to take their feelings into account.

How do you tell the extended family?

Once we knew the truth about what was the matter with Matt we had to think about how we would explain it to the family, which was one of the hardest battles. We had different types of reaction from them. Some of them were quite accepting;

others seemed to take the view that any special needs children should be in homes, which was very upsetting. You do have to remember that an older generation may struggle to accept the idea of a condition that was not recognised in their time, especially when their grandchild looks perfectly normal. All the grandparents found it hard to accept at first. It has taken a long time for them to see that Matt is different, not just naughty, but now they accept him for the person he is.

For a while we felt we couldn't take Matt anywhere within the family because of the way they reacted. A lot of the family found his condition baffling until they had learned more about it. Keith's Dad has a particularly good bond with Matt and understands his anxieties and needs. He drives him to school and is very considerate, trying to stick to the familiar routes, and letting Matt beep the horn on the corners. Matt is convinced that this is what you are supposed to do, so he gets cross if it isn't done. My Mum is good about understanding his communication problems, and will repeat sentences when he needs. All his grandparents find it easier now that Matt is older and they can clearly see that he is different from his peers and that he faces a lot of problems. His cousins, too, know him for who he is and will look out for him, which is great as I will not always be here and I want him to be able to live normally but know he can get help if he needs it from people who care about him. His brothers and sister all know how he will need them later on in life. The special bond makes them a stronger family unit and I feel I have done well here.

- You need support from your family – be honest and try to make them understand what they can do to help you.

- Tell your other children sooner rather than later.
- Find a support group if at all possible and talk to others in the same position as you. In the first instance contact the NAS Autism Helpline (0845 0704004).
- Investigate local sibling support groups (we were referred by our paediatrician) and try to find one for the right age range for your children.
- There will be behaviour that upsets siblings: be prepared to help them understand and deal with it.
- Timetable in time to be with your other children – they need you too.
- If you feel that your child would like to have friends, be pro-active in helping establish bonds with other children.
- Investigate the possibilities for respite care – it will help you to restore some balance in the family. Use the time to do family things and ask your other children what they would like to do.
- Go to talks on autism and learn about it.
- It is not the end of the world. Try to be happy with it yourself.

How does the situation affect your friendships?

I found it hard at diagnosis. Some friends accepted it and were supportive, some – not the ones I would have expected – cut me off. It hurt when I felt that I had lost some friends at such a personally vulnerable time. Some friends we have now are very fond of Matt and accept the way he is, so we are relaxed when they are around, and Matt's godmother is a tower of strength.

What is awful to start with is that tense feeling with your child when you are out, wondering if he will behave, or what he will do next – like a toddler time-bomb but **all** the time. It does make you tense and defensive, but as you get more used to it you do find out what works and what doesn't as far as social life is concerned. It is best to compromise a bit and not put yourself under pressure to keep your old life as it was.

The boys went through a stage where they were embarrassed to bring friends home because of Matt, but as they have got older they have learned to deal with his behaviour and now they tell mates before they arrive at the house, 'my brother is different, don't be offended if he says something odd – he's a great guy but he is not like us.'

How can friends help?

Most of our friends just accept that this is the way we are as a family. I have a good friend who I can always chat to when I need a sympathetic ear. She listens and we can have a joke about things. She doesn't judge me as a parent but will always help. What you need is support not advice. Sometimes, when I feel a bit overwhelmed, she drags me out for a girly evening, which does me a power of good. Some friends have built up a rapport with Matt and take him for the day, though with some people it is too much worry.

Real friends will not judge you or your family. You know who they are, but remember it can sometimes be difficult for even good friends to understand as they do not go through this each day like us.

- As a good friend, don't get upset if the child says something hurtful like 'I don't like your dress' –understand that he really doesn't mean to be rude.
- Be patient with the child.
- Be a good listener.
- Understand that all days are not the same.
- Don't judge the rest of the family because of this child.
- Volunteer to go with your friend who has an ASD child to meetings with health professionals and teachers, write down what they are saying and talk it through afterwards. Sometimes it is just too much for one person to take in on her own, and moral support is wonderful.

Can you help an ASD child to be more sociable?

The level of contact Matt has is not typical of Asperger's sufferers, but right from the start I have helped him to socialise. When they said at nursery that he wasn't socialising, I felt that he had to have friends and we would have to help him get them. Having older brothers was the key because they would bring friends round and that meant that Matt could see the relationships and thought he would like the same for himself. So, when he started school, I invited children to tea so they could see him at home and it progressed from there. At first he couldn't face talking to other children, but he learned how to through his brothers.

- Have family meals and be strict about making your ASD child do his best to join in – he is part of the family, and this is a first step towards an outside social life.
- When he finds it hard, get the others to go at his pace and let him talk without interruption.
- Help him to want to interact with other people by teaching him some useful social skills, such as how to join in a conversation, where to stand and so on.
- Encourage him to play with other children – board games (perhaps with a sympathetic adult at first while he gets the idea) and outdoor games and activities such as trampolining.
- Join cubs, swimming clubs, drama or music groups – it all helps.

What about unsuitable friendships?

Matt is very different from some Asperger's people in that he is sociable and he loves his friends, but unfortunately the children he mixes with are very outgoing and game for a laugh, and sometimes they exploit his condition. They will suggest something and he will go off and do it, which can land him in trouble. I do worry about what they get up to but, on the other hand, I am glad he has friends. You can try to channel your child into a different direction with friendships, but ultimately, if you want them to have friends there is only so much you can do. You can try to socialise as much as possible with your child to push them in the direction of more suitable friendships, or find other children with the same interests. But you might come across some parents who will not let their child play with yours.

What can you do when a parent loses his or her temper with the child?

As a family we help each other. If someone dealing with Matt is starting to lose it we hand over to someone else. You do more harm than good if you try to stick it out with him as you raise his anxiety, which leads to bigger problems.

- If you feel you are losing it call time out for yourself. If you are on your own then say you will be back in ten minutes and go to the bathroom just to cool off. When you return you will be able to see the problem more clearly as you will have had time to think.
- So that the child doesn't think he has won you say to him, with your hand up, 'not discussing'. It is important for both of you that you are still in charge of the situation.

How can people outside the family cope with your child?

- Be patient!
- If you are left to look after the child it is most likely that you know him fairly well already, so plan ahead a bit and think of things you know he likes to do.
- Know how to use the PECs picture symbols, if that is how he communicates, and make sure you know what the house

rules and regulations are – this is important with any child, vital with ASD children.

- Remember to talk straight to the child, saying his name clearly first.

Chapter 5

Coping emotionally and getting support

Bringing up a child with an autistic spectrum disorder has many rewards but, make no mistake, it can be a relentlessly draining process. You need a lot of support from family and friends, and even then, a short break from time to time may be the best thing for you and your family. For this reason, I am going to write at length about respite care at this point, because it has made all the difference to my family.

Respite care can be a lifeline

When Matt was eight the social services said we could have respite and when I asked the children what they thought about it they said 'does that mean we could have a normal weekend just with you?' That clinched it, really. Respite brought the closeness back – I hadn't realised quite how much our family life had been compromised.

Respite care involves Matt going to someone else for one long weekend a month. It has made a huge difference to our family, and has been a crucial step in restoring some balance to our family life, and giving the other children the attention they needed. It meant that I could do things with them to make up for all the time when I was concentrating on Matt. I felt I needed to have some time with the other children just to have an uninterrupted chat. We would go out for walks and just do things on the spur of the moment, which is normally impossible, and if we wanted to play a game we could without Matt disrupting it. Such simple things, but they have always meant a lot to us. We really need that precious family time when we can just relax.

Matt used to accept the respite care fantastically. As he has got older he doesn't like it so much but we keep it going because the other children need it. I think in a way it will help him to mature because it is good for him to have to make the effort with someone who isn't family and to accept that things are different at another house. He has always been to the same person and if I have to be in hospital (I am asthmatic and have spinal problems for which I have had seven operations) I can call her and she will take him so he doesn't have to go somewhere that he doesn't know, which wouldn't work for him at all. It is definitely worth trying to set up an arrangement like this if you can, and you should be able to do so through the social services.

Initially I felt very inadequate to be asking for help, as if it meant that I couldn't cope as a mother, but unless you live with a child like Matt you can't really appreciate the stresses of the situation. It is hard as a parent to say, 'I can't cope.' I made myself say it in the mirror and somehow saying it to myself like that made a difference. I think that in some ways it is a sign of strength to be able to acknowledge that you need some help and it is better for the whole family if you decide to get what you can. When I first spoke to a social worker she asked if I wanted Matt put into foster care. Of course, nothing was further from my mind: all I was asking for was respite, which is not the same at all. My advice to anyone who thinks that respite care might be the answer is to speak to your key worker about it and keep trying. Don't be put off if you have a long wait.

I have established an excellent relationship with Zena, Matt's carer, and we have a continuity of care between us. She will reinforce any discipline that I have tried to establish and she will have Matt sometimes at short notice when I really need a break. She comes with me to Matt's reviews at school and gives me a lot of support – she is much more than simply respite to us.

Parents fall into a trap if they feel that they are the only ones who can possibly have a special relationship with their child, it can be so beneficial to have another adult who is involved. I can understand how parents get so stressed if they are coping alone. Help should be forthcoming straight away if parents need it, though of course it often isn't. You shouldn't be put on a waiting list when you are desperate.

Under the new system of direct payments you are given a set amount of money a month to spend on respite and on other beneficial things like someone to take your child shopping or on outings to the cinema or things like music lessons.

As Matt gets older his needs are changing from the one-to-one respite care to things that are more socially inclined and outward looking. He can have a paid companion to help him in case things go wrong as he takes steps out into the wider world and learns how to do things for himself. He can also have someone paid to give him help with his homework. The money is there and you decide how best it can be used for your child. Then at age 16, he should be able to take control of it himself and at 18 he definitely can.

Zena Fisher has been Matt's respite carer since he was eight. 'I work at a special school as well. My parents were respite carers and they looked after very severely disabled children so the work held no fears for me. I have been a respite carer for 13 years and currently have 10 children slotted in at different times: they entertain and play with each other and it is good for the less able ones to be with more able children. The able ones do become more caring. It builds up their self-esteem and Matt is very good with the less able children. You need to have a very open, honest relationship with the parents for respite to work well – the kind of relationship where you can tell each other if something isn't going right. After a while they all become part of your extended family. My daughter who is eight thinks this is just normal family life because she has never known any different and I am sure that she and her friends will grow up as much more rounded adults because of their experience.

'I am respite carer for four people with Asperger's and they are all different. It is important to remember that, apart from having the same idiosyncrasies, they have their own personalities. Different things trigger them and you can't have too many preconceived rules when you are caring for them. You can expect too much from people who are good at communicating, and, with Asperger's, they do not look at all disabled so people can have unrealistic expectations. That is one of the challenges for the children and the parents.'

Different types of respite care

Various kinds of care are available to help you, most of which require local authority funding and not all of which are available to everyone. You can find out more from your local social services.

1. Home-based respite care.
2. Family-based short-term respite, which is similar to foster care. A disabled child is matched with a family and then stays with them on a regular basis.
3. Children's homes which offer residential short-term care which gives respite to families.
4. After-school activities, youth clubs, play schemes and summer camps.
5. Residential schools.
6. Befriending schemes run by the National Autistic Society through its volunteering network (0115 911 3369 for details).

Dealing with everyday stress

When I have had a really bad day and snap at Matt then my husband takes over when he gets home so I can shut off for a while. I try to make sure I have an hour a day to relax away from all the constant questions and so on. I think it is very important to get a break, the relentlessness of the condition can be exhausting for carers and that is why it can be so much harder for single parents if they don't have anyone else who can take over for a while.

Time-table some stress-relief

One thing that can help you long term is to make a note of which parts of the day are most stressful for you, perhaps by making a chart that you fill in every day for a while. If all the family members do this, you will fairly quickly be able to see which parts of the day are the low points, and try to organise extra help, perhaps from extended family and friends, at these times. Perhaps grandpa can give the children a lift to an evening activity, or a friend can sit with your ASD child for an hour while you go to yoga – anything that stops you from feeling you are being split in two by the additional demands of the situation.

- Make sure you get a chance to relax when the children have all gone to bed – a long soak in the bath, a glass of wine, an outing with a friend – you deserve a reward and this is your time.
- This can be harder for single parents, but do what you can – phone someone for a chat, or get a friend to come round to you.
- Sign up for a Home-Start helper to give you a morale boost.

Safeguarding relationships and coping as parents

Your relationship with your partner is very special and you need to make sure you have time for yourselves. Looking after your family, and in particular your ASD child, is a very demanding job, and you need a break from time to time, in this job more than most. Here are a few tips to think about:

- Go out for a meal together or have a special meal at home with no interruptions.
- Find a babysitter you can trust so you can relax when you are out.
- Go on a picnic or for a walk together when the children are at school.
- If you are lucky with family who will look after the kids then have a few days away – just the two of you.

You both need time together, if you don't make time you will risk the rows happening and this is no good for you or your family. If you are a single parent, you need some relaxation time even more. Don't ever be too proud to ask family and friends for help, and for their time.

The mixed emotions you have as a parent of a child with special needs are awful; guilt haunts you. There are lots of trigger points. I felt very low at first when we had the diagnosis, but I knew I had to square up to it, and I did. Keith found it incredibly hard. Matt was his first child. He was devastated and blamed himself and it took him a long time to come to terms with it. I was the one who went to all the meetings and the talks and told him what I had learned. Mostly it was the Mums at the meetings. Most men find that sort of thing really hard, but Keith did think it was comforting that there were other Dads like him.

Parents go through a stage of blaming themselves. In the end you just have to accept that this thing has happened. You get situations where the mother can't cope and the child goes into care or the father just walks away. The feelings of isolation are hard to bear. Support is crucial at this time. Be aware that it is not unusual to have irrational feelings of shame.

Sometimes you almost feel you are being victimised because you have had this child. That is so wrong: it is hard enough to accept that your child is different without having to fight for everything you need. Every person with children like this misses support and understanding from family when it is not there, but all the difficulties made Keith and I feel our relationship was stronger than it was before. I could see where the pitfalls could break a relationship, and in fact a high percentage of marriages where a child in the family has special needs do break up.

Any condition that affects the mind is still a big taboo in parts of our society. I have been at the school gates waiting to pick Matt up when another parent has come up to me and said 'I don't wish my child to catch what yours has so I don't want him anywhere near.' I did not bother to reply to this breathtaking ignorance but it still left me embarrassed and upset. On another day we were having lunch when we were shopping and Matt had an epileptic fit. A woman came up to us and said 'it puts me off my food; you should not bring a child like that out.' It just made me despair.

As a parent you have to accept that your child is different, and this can take time. Once you have grieved over the loss of a normal, healthy child you can start again. Parents do need some time to come to terms with everything. Don't rush it, you need to understand the situation you are in yourself, then you can see what you can do to help. I soon found my feet when putting my energy into helping Matt. Now I am so proud of my family but most of all I am proud of Matt as he has come so far.

- Give yourselves time to come to terms with the situation, this is a hard time and you need to square up to it.
- Don't be too proud to ask for help and support.
- Contact a Family is a nationwide charity giving advice, information and support to parents of disabled children and helping parents to contact other families locally and nationally. Helpline 0808 808 3555 **www.cafamily.org.uk**.

Chapter 6

Communication

A Lego™ game will make you think

If we always remember the need to explain things to our ASD children it might make life much easier. There is an exercise we did in my training that I think everyone should try. Two people each have the same little Lego ™ set to assemble, but they cannot see each other. One has to assemble the set using only the instructions they are given verbally by the other. I will be amazed if anyone gets this right first time. It just shows how difficult it can be to communicate everything to another person. You have to explain all the things you normally do automatically; you have to explain each and every step of the way. Once you have tried it you will realise how much we constantly assume that other people know, and you just can't do that with a child with ASD.

If you try this game yourself, be exact in your definitions, and keep remembering to say the other person's name, so he knows you are talking to him. This leads me on to some of the golden rules for :

Communicating with your ASD child

- Use the child's name repeatedly – they need to know that you are talking to them.

Get the child's full attention and try to exclude background noise like the television so they can concentrate on you.

- Use simple language with no unnecessary words and say exactly what you mean – no fancy turns of phrase such as 'I'm hopping mad' or 'I laughed my head off' – remember these children are very literal-minded.
- Allow them the time they need to understand what you have said and process information.
- Give the child a reason to communicate, so that they can get something they want, whether it is food or a toy that you have put out of reach. From a very early age I got Matt to say what he wanted, not just point to it, so before he could have what he wanted he had to make an effort.
- Be definite in what you say, especially when it is about the time you will do things. 'We will go out straight after breakfast', or 'you can watch television at 5 o'clock'.
- Use picture symbols or photos to communicate if that is easier for them (see chapter 2).
- Be positive and tell them what they **should** be doing rather than what they shouldn't.
- Only promise things you can deliver.

I have learned quite a lot through doing specialised courses, and if parents have the time I recommend that they do the same. You can get details of courses from your local library or Further Education college or from the NAS website **www.autism.org.uk**.

I used to work as a veterinary assistant and what sticks in my mind with my approach to Matt is how you train a dog. Those simple, straightforward instructions: 'sit, now', 'stay, now' were what we were limited to. With most children you assume they know certain things, with dogs you assume they know nothing, so that approach is not as daft as it sounds. It worked with Matt, and it still works. 'Matt, hand, hold, now!' works, where something more complex, abstract and confusing to him does not.

Tones of voice

Your child needs to understand that you will use different tones of voice for different situations.

1. Normal voice when talking.
2. Voice of authority, which is firm, for when they need control/discipline.
3. Calming voice, lower than usual, to help them out of a tantrum or panic.

How to help your child develop conversation skills

- Give them lots of practice in how to start a conversation and then keep it going.
- Get them used to the idea of changing topics, and not holding forth at length on something that they find fascinating.
- Teach them not to talk for too long – perhaps you could practise with an egg timer.

Chapter 7

Behaviour

'That child needs a good slap!'

'That mother should be ashamed of herself letting him behave like that!'

Prepare to harden your heart; your child's behaviour is likely to bring out the intolerant worst in a lot of people. Of course, they don't know what they are talking about, or what you have to go through every day, and if they did I hope they would not be so quick to judge. Don't worry about what other people think. The important thing is that you deal with behaviour that you find a problem in a way that works for you and your child. I have found the best way to cope with things is by not moving boundaries. A child with ASD likes to walk a firm black line – that is what feels safe. If the child goes into a grey area, anxiety increases and you end up with a bigger problem. The important thing is that your rules have to stay the same at all times, no matter how hard this is to do. That way your child feels safe and you are in control.

Helping them to change bad habits

- Work out what you wish to change and why.

- Plan how you are going to do it.
- Explain to them why and how they need to change.
- Ask the family to help – if you are all consistent you can avoid giving crossed messages.
- Reward good habits – and when they have **tried** to stop doing something bad
- Have goals they can reach.
- Make a reward chart together, so it can feature treats that relate to whatever they are into at the time.

Our aim is always to make sure that Matt really understands what we are trying to do. Sometimes if we go over things two or three times that will be enough; sometimes we may be repeating something for months or years on end. If he digs his heels in straight away, we know we are in for a battle. In that case, the key is to see what is making him angry or confused. I write everything down and sometimes I can see that I have missed out one thing in the sequence of what he has to do, and that means the whole thing doesn't work for him because he can't understand it.

- Assess your behaviour as well as theirs. Do you explain things in enough detail?

Flapping

Matt used to flap and shake his hands, as if he was frantically fanning his face with both hands. The need to flap is common among people with ASDs, along with similar repetitive self-stimulatory habits, known collectively as 'stimming'. Some-times they do it through anxiety, sometimes through habit, sometimes for comfort. I usually found with Matt that he did it when he was anxious, and if he was left to it, it would lead into rocking, which always looked very disturbing.

If you have a child in a playground flapping his arms then other children would stare and be frightened, or puzzled, or amused, and in the same way, when you have a young man buying drinks at a bar and flapping his arms, they are quite likely to think he has had enough to drink already and refuse to serve him. None of these responses are what you want for your child when you are trying to integrate them into the world, so we wanted to modify the flapping to something a bit less conspicuous.

We developed this routine where I would just put my hand up, which was the stop signal, say 'stop' gently but firmly in a low voice and then say 'tap' and he would copy me and move his hands down to tap his leg instead, and then gradually we changed it to tapping his side. I wasn't taking his flapping away from him altogether but replacing it with another habit that was easier to cope with. He still taps on his side now, when he feels the need to, but it is not as obvious as somebody flapping their arms. He is still being allowed to flap or tap but it doesn't look so distinctive or odd to other people. It doesn't now have the look of something that people would see and judge him for. The tapping is much calmer and doesn't fuel his anxiety like the flapping did. Interestingly, when we got him out of the flapping habit, he stopped rocking, too. The whole thing has become much less extreme for him.

Flapping by Matthew Keith Brealy

'I am glad my mum stopped me flapping because I would look like an abnormal kid and my mates would not like it.'

The reason that you might want to modify extreme habits is just so that your ASD child won't look so different in a society that is not very tolerant of difference. There is no reason that they should have to fit in with our society, but they will probably have a better time if they don't stand out from the crowd too much. This sort of modification will give them the best chance to fit in. It can take a very long time to establish. It took us 12 to 18 months to work on Matt's flapping to the point where it was hardly happening at all. You can't get someone with an ASD to stop doing things like that completely, because these habits are part of the way they meet the world, and also a relief for them.

When Matt does the replacement activity he gets the same degree of comfort out of it, which is important. A lot of people tap on the side of their leg in time to music or whatever, so he won't stand out too much. For us, it has been a slow, gentle modification. When you are trying to get your child to do something like this, which takes constant repetition of an instruction from you, you have to keep calm, and keep your voice very low and gentle, every time, and say something reassuring, like 'it's ok, you can bring your hands down, we can tap together'.

If other parents got cross or agitated when they were trying to deal with something like the flapping, then they would probably make it worse, and the child would do it all the more. All you are doing then is giving them even more anxiety, because they won't understand why you are saying 'stop'. These habits are important to ASD sufferers. They tend to like things like twiddling a pen, so, if you are teaching them, you give them a card for 'twiddle time' if they seem to need it. Give them five minutes off class work and then they know they are going back to work afterwards. So they still get things done, and if it is at a slower rate, what does it matter?

Tantrums

People with ASDs all have different habits, and there are some things you simply have to try to stop. If your child is having a tantrum on the floor, you go down to their level and in a very calm voice you hold out your hand and say 'five, four, three, two, one, finished now, let's go and do something else'. So you have taken them away from what was making them panicky – if they wanted to play with a ball or something else that wasn't there – just by doing that and changing the focus. You have stopped the tantrum calmly and quietly given them something else to think about. Then say something like 'Okay, you can have five minutes with the ball and then we are going to do something else'. Then give them an egg timer and time it. When the time is up you do something else, just like you said you would. A lot of these techniques work really well with neurotypical children as well.

It helps your child, when he has got in a state, to have a familiar format. You are his safety net; if you get angry and move your boundaries around, he will get confused and he won't feel safe. If you keep the boundaries the same and say very firmly that you have asked him to finish his tantrum, then you have taken over where he has lost control, and he feels safe because you have told him what he is going to do and that it is something that he can manage. So you take his mind off what the tantrum was – you tell him that you are going to paint now, or to play with a ball, and then you can deal with what caused the tantrum in the beginning. Maybe he was trying to do something that frustrated him because it was too difficult or beyond his age range.

Your strength is very reinforcing for your child, so you have to make sure that you can be strong. You have to stay calm with him all the time, even if inside you feel as if you are about to flip your lid. I have sometimes had to go into a different room and scream.

This type of behaviour often gets lumped under the heading of 'challenging behaviour' but I think that is entirely the wrong definition. ASD tantrums or panics are invariably a response to things that your child feels have gone out of control, an expression of unhappiness and fear. I would call challenging behaviour something that is pro-active, and seeks a response – of course, you will probably have to deal with both types of behaviour from time to time.

ASD children do sometimes communicate emotions in a way that seems violent. They will generally only hit out as a response when something is bothering them. I do not think that this is challenging behaviour, just a basic reaction. A child with ASD could virtually strangle someone, not for any malicious reason but because they wanted to shut them up.

What to do if noise causes tantrums and anxiety

Matt would sometimes have tantrums when we were just sitting watching television, and it was hard to understand why. In the end I realised that he just couldn't bear loud noises and the tantrums always started when there was something like a police siren on television, and when that happened, he just wouldn't stay in the room. We tried to protect him from loud noises while we got him used to them so that they wouldn't cause him such problems.

We would always stay indoors on firework night because Matt really hated all the noise. Gradually, over a long time, we got as far as watching the fireworks on the doorstep and then, after even longer, we could watch them outside without Matt freaking out.

We helped Matt deal with the fear of noises by getting him to make loud noises himself, playing with pots and pans and, later, his brother's drum kit. Matt is much better about noise now. Reacting to his problems and changing what **we** do rather than trying to change what **he** feels has always been our best way of coping.

The art of dealing with noise:

- Try playing music games.
- Take them to music therapy to get them used to different types of noise.

- Go to the fire station and look at the fire engines – ask them to put on a siren if they are not too busy.
- Play at being police cars – crime fighting can get really noisy.

Incentives for good behaviour

- Choose incentives to help your child behave. If they are obsessed with a particular video, for instance, let them watch it when they have behaved well.
- One incentive that seems to work well for us is this: Matt gets £1 a night if he is where he should be at the right time, but he loses £1 if he isn't. The same principle applies if we want him to behave better at school. He gets £1 for a praise card from school, and loses £1 for a bad report.

The Golden Rules

Another idea that is used a lot in school, and would work at home, too, is the 'golden rules'. These are behaviour points that are set out firmly in the class, and children are rewarded for their compliance. I made up my own set to use with Matt, which are aimed at autistic children, and you could make up your own to suit your child.

Matt is gentle	Matt does not hurt anyone
Matt will listen to people	Matt will not interrupt
Matt will put his toys away	Matt will not leave his toys for someone else to tidy

Matt will try hard at school	Matt will not walk out of school
Matt is kind to others	Matt will not hurt the feelings of others

What you can do when behaviour is a problem

- Use simple instructions – make sure they have really understood.
- Stay calm – especially when dealing with tantrums – if you get angry it will make ASD sufferers very anxious.
- If your child is clearly getting angry or upset, try to get them to go out to the garden or somewhere else that is safe – and make it easy for them to get there without too much in their way.
- Stick to your guns. Be consistent with your rules and make sure that others who look after your child do the same. Stick to punishments you impose – even if it makes you miserable.
- Say to the child 'this is unacceptable behaviour, we do not hit Fred/ bite Jemima', etc. Say that they will be punished if they continue the unacceptable behaviour. Always use the same format of words.
- Remember that a lot of what seems like bad behaviour is rooted in anxiety – can you work out what might be making them anxious? Is there a medical reason such as toothache or a headache?
- Listen to your child – when they are upset they may be trying to tell you something. See if there is a pattern to their behaviour.

- Don't move the boundaries – it will make them feel unsafe.
- Be prepared for it to take a long time to modify habits.
- Be sure that the child understands what they have done wrong, but remember that they are not very likely to learn from experience. You have to go over and over again how **not** to do something. Matt promises he will not do things again, but if someone says 'try this,' he always will.
- Remember that you are their safety net when they are in a tantrum; you provide the boundaries that make them feel secure.
- Keep your voice low and calm – go into a different room to scream!

To punish or not to punish?

All punishment has to be done as soon as the child has misbehaved or they will not know why they are being punished. Keep explaining again and again why you are doing this. Say 'well done' when they have completed the punishment, so they get a better understanding that the punishment has finished and it is time to move on.

- As an effective method of punishment I have tried taking away something Matt values for a short time. I put the egg timer on to show how long the punishment is for and so that he can see it is not forever.
- With some older children, grounding can be effective, but you have to explain how it works each time you do this, and why you are grounding them.

Preventing dangerous behaviour

If your ASD child is doing something dangerous and you have to stop them quickly, getting cross doesn't help. You can shout and it won't have any effect because they can't see why you are getting cross. They don't understand the dangers we see. I have learned through Matt that what you have to do is explain over and over again why things are dangerous. For instance, with a fire, you show him pictures of some of the bad things that could happen, and that helps him to understand. ASD children still find the concept of cause and effect very hard to grasp, and you have to go over and over and over what may happen if they do whatever it is. Even now, Matt will still do things that he doesn't realise are dangerous, so we have to go over and over it with him: 'this is what could happen if you don't stop at a junction on your bike,' and then show him an awful picture of an accident, because maybe that will sink in.

- Try to understand why the child is behaving this way – has something triggered the situation? Can you remove it or make it easier for next time?
- Remember that it is very likely that these children are working very hard to keep a lid on all their feelings during the school day, so by the time they get home they are just about ready to explode. You have to understand the level of stress they are coping with.
- Ask yourself if their anxiety levels are high and, if so, why?
- If you can find out what is making them unhappy, you will see why they are behaving badly.

- If their behaviour is dangerous, explain why they cannot do this, and, if you can, show them what the outcome could be.
- Channel them into something different.
- Talk to them about what makes them cross – remove it if you can, or try between you to find an acceptable way round it.
  - Matt would wind people up because he liked to see their faces go red when he did. Accepting authority is hard for these children; they can't see why adults should tell children what to do, and yet they need the safety of discipline and structure.

Helping them to calm down

If the child is trying to do an activity and is getting anxious about it, then change how you do the activity. If the child is anxious because of something in the room, remove the child for five to ten minutes as a break. This should happen at your command. So you are saying 'let's do something else,' and then you can bring them back at the point where their anxiety levels have gone down and you can start again.

If they lose it totally they need to let off steam, so let them. Then go in and in a calm, low voice say '5,4,3,2,1, time out.' Then they have time out in a room where they can be quiet. You have helped them get over the anxiety and move on. You are the safety net. But, of course, you aren't always there. And it is important that they have some things they can do for themselves.

Teaching them how to calm themselves down

I have taught Matt that if a teacher, or someone else, is shouting and he doesn't like it, he should imagine that the words are just floating right over his head. Matt says that this helps him a lot.

Sometimes Matt will put his hand up and say 'I need time out' and this kind of awareness, which comes before an anxiety state or tantrum can set in, is what we are aiming for.

Matt used to hold all his tension in all day at school and smile and get through the day and then explode when he got home. Some children will explode like this just anywhere, depending on the severity of their condition. Matt always seemed to know instinctively how to hold his feelings in until he got home – most of the time at least. He would be anxious as soon as I picked him up from school – you could see it in his body – and as soon as he got home he would keep saying 'time out'. He had to be left alone in his room for two hours and then he would come out and have tea and be fine. If he got interrupted, he would just explode and trash his room. He would smash a toy that he loved and at first he wouldn't make the connection that his rage had broken it and it would have to be thrown out – and he hates throwing things away. Matt feels he can control a tantrum himself now, where it used to be me saying 'you need time out' and taking him to his room. We have had to respect his need for time out. It is his safety net. He still goes over the top sometimes, but much less now because he knows how to control himself.

He has a 'time out' card at school, too, because otherwise he might throw a chair or something. If he gets into a state where he cannot cope in class, he gets the card and the teacher lets him go off to the special needs teacher's room, where he has a soft drink, calms himself down and talks it through. Then we can analyse what triggered it – if the work was too hard, or there was something he didn't understand. Whatever it was, we can use the information for next time. It removes him from doing what he didn't want to do. Teachers are good about it – better a 'time out' card than a table in your face.

We have got Matt his own headset, which has really helped. His anxiety builds up when there is a lot of noise around and now he can listen to music on the headset to block out everything around him for a while – which reduces his anxiety levels. He can initiate that for himself, when it all gets too much, and now they have allowed him to have it in school as well, so he can switch off from the outside world, listen to music and come back again when he is ready.

- Find some techniques that work for your child – like imagining anger-inducing words floating over his head.
- Give him a 'time out' space at home and respect his need for it.
- Get his teacher to let him have a 'time out' card at school – and make sure the teacher understands that when it appears she must take it seriously.
- Listening to music on a headset can block out noise that he is finding too much and help him to calm down.

Getting cross by Matthew Keith Brealy

'I get frustrated when teachers or people don't believe me this gets me cross, I hate it when people talk too fast I get lost in what they are saying. This gets me cross too. I don't like it when I get pushed I want to hit them when they do this I say stop it. My Mum has shown me that when people shout to let the words go over my head I feel this works and helps to control my anger.'

Chapter 8

Changes and obsessions – trying to achieve flexibility of thought

Matthew's major obsession when he was younger was lining up his cars and Action men, which is a fairly textbook piece of behaviour. He would spend hours setting everything up and it had to be in exactly the right place. If I moved anything so much as a fraction he would notice in an instant and get very anxious. Among ASD children anxiety and panic attacks when we disrupt a pattern, or do something they don't understand, can cause behaviour that to an outsider looks like a violent tantrum, but in reality is anxiety that has gone off the scale.

When he was younger, Matt simply couldn't bear any deviation from routine and I realised that, for his own sake, we had to help him accept changes. Gradually, I started to make little changes to see how he would cope with them. I would put one of his toy cars round the wrong way and then I would say 'I like it that way round.' Then we would change another one together, and slowly he got the hang of changing things around. Then we took a really deep breath and repainted his room a different colour. Little by little he got used to changes like this and realised that they wouldn't hurt him

Ways to achieve flexibility of thought

The rigid clinging to routine is a big part of ASD, and can cause your child lots of extra problems in coping with a world that does not always oblige by sticking to patterns. You can really help if you encourage them to see that little things in their day can change without anything terrible happening. Show them the positive side – for instance, they do not have to bath at 8.00 pm sharp every day, they can finish watching their television programme first if they want to.

You really have to help them to learn flexibility of thought. For instance, if you need to change something little, let the child help. Explain what needs to happen and ask how they think it can be done. Do not do this unless your child can cope with it – you will know from him when the time is right. I was overjoyed when, one day, Matt volunteered that I should pick his sister up before him, which was a change to routine that really helped me out on that day. He coped with it really well, partly because it had been his idea. It may seem like a small thing, but for us it represented a massive step forward in Matt's way of thinking.

When something has to change in our daily routine, I tell Matt what the change is and why it is going to happen and what is going to happen instead, and go over it lots of times. Then, just before the change happens, I explain yet again. I know this seems incredibly long-winded but it is better than coping with a tantrum.

- Getting used to lots of insignificant little changes will help them to feel safer with the idea of change.

- Explain any change in routine to them lots of times before it happens.

Obsessive interests

Matt had a bit of an obsession with fires. It started, rather unfortunately, when a teacher asked him to find out the difference between flammable and inflammable for homework. Matt wasn't to know that it was a trick question and, predictably enough, took a very literal approach to his research. Once we had cleared up the mess in the kitchen, it became his great interest to continue this research long term, and he discovered that quite a lot of things are, actually, flammable (or indeed, inflammable). It was quite hard to get him to stop but, as we clearly had to get through to him before he burned the house down, I discovered that you can get a fireman to come to your home and explain the unwisdom of starting little experimental fires around the place. A fireman in full uniform is an impressive sight, and Matt took his message very much to heart. If you are having problems with an obsession it is worth looking for a simple and direct solution like this one.

Learning to throw things away

Matt has a big problem with throwing things away which I am trying to work on. Recently we went through his wardrobe and found things that were too small and that he didn't wear any more, so we put them in a big bag to take to the charity shop. The idea that they weren't going to be thrown out but handed on to someone who might need them seems okay with him, so we are getting him used to the idea of recycling. It is important, so that when he has somewhere of his own one day it won't be floor to ceiling with old shoes.

ASD people tend to be collectors and don't like changing things by getting rid of anything. This is a life-long characteristic and dealing with it is an important part of conforming to normal life. Potentially, you could end up with a house crammed with stuff. I knew one person who found it hard to get rid of the wrappers off her food – imagine the smell. Every time you threw something away the anxiety of someone like that would be enormous, so you need to address the problem as early as possible. With something like food containers, perhaps you could try washing them and making models out of them for a while and then getting rid of them. It is all part of getting ASD children used to things they don't like.

Transition

As we know, change of any kind is extremely hard for ASD children to cope with. When you know a change is coming up it will make things much easier if you do everything you can to ease the period of transition. Moving school, changing carers, moving house or any other major change is a very anxious time for ASD sufferers of any age. There is a lot we can do to help with this one, and I advise you do it!

- If moving school, ask if your child could do some extra familiarisation days in the school the week before they start. This will break them in slowly without the huge number of children starting on the same day and gives them the advantage of getting to know their way around the school a bit before the others arrive.

- Ask if you can both meet the new teacher together.
- Ask if you could have photos of the teachers who will be teaching your child. Take the pictures home and let the child get used to their faces. Remember to put the teachers' names at the bottom of each picture for an extra bit of familiarisation.
- Go over the route to school if it is new, using a map if you need to.
- Use a calendar to make a count down to the day when school will start.
- If changing to a new carer, get a picture of him or her and cross the days off on the calendar till the old carer will leave and the new one will start.
- When moving house, take the child to the house to see all the rooms and to explore the new place.
- Count down to the move date.
- Show the child his new room.
- Show the child the route to the new house.

Make yourself some notes on how you dealt with any particular change; what helped and what didn't. You will find the notes really useful to refer back to next time a similar situation arises.

Bereavement and loss

A person with ASD will encounter many losses in their time, as for them the loss of a pen or a favourite item may well have the same significance as the loss of a person. You need to be ready for this and talk to them about replacing the lost item, which, ideally, they should choose. In the case of bereavement of a person you will need to have a long talk and explain the individual situation. When a person they are involved with in everyday life, such as a carer, is leaving, do the count-downs and charts described above. This prevents your child from having a huge build-up of anxiety and, once again, you are preparing them for a change, which they would find it hard to cope with unaided.

Chapter 9

Strategies for dealing with day-to-day difficulties

Your ASD child sees most things in a different way to the rest of the family and, if left to himself – well, there is no point going down that road because, however much some of them might like it, they probably couldn't really be left to themselves. So, you have to fit everybody together so that life can run along reasonable lines. Nobody said it would be easy – but there are ways of dealing with a lot of daily challenges.

- Don't look for a miracle cure – work realistically to deal with what you have.
- Keeping a written record helps you to see patterns of behaviour.
- Camcording behaviour can help. It is easier to understand what causes particular situations when you look at them from a calm distance and then you can deal with them.
- Look for a strategy in each situation.
- See if you are eligible for any grants that will help you to modify your house so that you can cope better.
- Respect your child's routines and need for sameness – for instance at bedtime.

- Doing things they way they like will really help them, so if you want to change something do it carefully.
- Adapting to his needs makes your life easier.

Sleep problems

When Matt was very young he didn't sleep and he was in and out of bed many, many times a night. That is very typical behaviour for ASD children. They don't seem to settle, they can't switch off and they quite often suffer from night terrors; scary, waking type dreams which are as disturbing for onlookers as they are for the sufferer. Matt would dream of things that he thought were really there – often it was snakes on the floor. At first we didn't know what to make of it. He was petrified. I would sit down and talk to him and calm him down. Sometimes we would have a hot drink and then we would go back and try to go to sleep again.

Taking our time seemed to work better than just putting the light on to show him there was nothing there and then going back to sleep. If we did that, a few minutes later he would be up again with the same thing. He needed us to spend that time with him to reassure him that everything was all right, and then get him back to sleep. If you put more time in yourself, you are more likely to get longer to sleep.

We actually did a video of Matt at night once to show the paediatrician how bad it was, and that was when he diagnosed night terrors. The camcorder helped us to look at the problem in the light of day and get some idea of how to deal with it.

That approach has helped with all sorts of things with Matt 's behaviour. I have always tried to look at what he was doing and write it all down. Being slightly removed from a situation helps you to see it more clearly and I find it is often easier to see why he is acting in a particular way when I think about it later.

If you are tired at night, the last thing you want is to start thinking about what to do, but if you already have a plan in place it really helps in the middle of the night. That is not the time for strategy forming. Camcording, taking notes and watching helped us to understand what was going on and to make a plan. It is much easier now, although Matt still gets the terrors from time to time. When this happens we take our time over the routine of going in, turning the light on, showing him there is nothing there and encouraging him to go back to sleep. We open the door, put more light into his room, we have a few regular things that reassure him and show him that he is all right.

If Matt's anxiety is raised in the day, we may have terrors in the night – it is all about unfinished business. He shouts and screams and walks about touching things. In the morning he has no idea that it happened. He is tired, but he has no idea why. Bits of what he remembers from his dream will come out in conversation during the day. We have tried to talk to him about it but he never remembers anything. He may have been up wandering around all night, but as far as he is concerned he was in bed asleep. It can be a big problem for the family.

Strategy for winding down in the evening:

- Start calming them down at least an hour before bed so they have time to unwind.
- Try using lavender oil in the room if they like it, this has a calming effect.
- Hot milky drinks work for some.
- Watch a calming favourite video, read a story, play together calmly with a favourite toy.
- Do all of these things together unless your child is happier alone. If you are together then you can check they are calming down.

Matt used to disturb the others. All three boys were in a bedroom together and the other two couldn't sleep through his night terrors, so were really tired for school the next morning. Sometimes he would do things like getting out of bed and hitting them with toys, pulling their duvets off, swapping things from bed to bed, moving things around. The upshot was that they just weren't sleeping and we were ending up with three grumpy boys in the morning instead of just one.

It was going from bad to worse, so, when I found out that I could get a grant towards getting another bedroom built in the attic, we were overjoyed. The older boys were able to move upstairs, where they could get their sleep undisturbed, and Matt moved into the small room next to us so that we could keep an eye on him.

Bedtime was always a problem for Matt. We would put him to

bed and he would be in and out sometimes till 11 or 12 at night, sometimes later, and then we were up I don't know how many times in the night. With bedtime we always had to stick to exactly the same routine. We had to check the windows, the curtains, under the bed, the duvet cover had to be right, the sheet had to be right, and all that still happens now. We found it better that one of us did it rather than both, so my husband made the routine where he goes in every single night.

Even now when Matt is 14, he won't go to bed unless his Dad puts him to bed and makes sure that everything is right. The curtains have to be just so and he knows if they are not right. Keith has to check under the bed and put the sheets right to tuck him in. He settles much quicker if everything is right. We have a respect for what he needs.

In some houses they might start saying 'this is ridiculous at his age' and try to make him conform to a more normal pattern, but we feel that respecting him as him is a key to helping him. Our long-term aim is that Matt would like to be able to put himself to bed, and we are working towards it bit by bit. So we do one less thing for him every so often until he has conquered that part of the routine for himself. We think it will take about 12-18 months for Matt to achieve independence in this area.

- Doing things the way ASD children like them is an important way to help them, so if you do need to change something do it very carefully.

Matt used to get very anxious if I so much as changed his duvet cover, because he always looked at the pattern when he was going to sleep and having the same shape, colour and pattern was very important to him. We got him to choose his own duvet covers so that he could make sure that they had a pattern he was comfortable with, and now, whenever I change it, it is to one he likes. By adapting to his needs we make our own lives easier as well.

When we went on holiday, sleep was an issue for him and he was worried. He actually wanted to dismantle his bed and take it with us, so we took his duvet instead, which made him feel secure and relaxed once we had made him understand that we had no room to take the whole bed. Then he felt settled because, with his duvet on the holiday bed, it looked like his bed at home. The look of things, the shapes, the patterns are very important to people with ASD.

Matt used to get up early and roam around the house but now he is reassuringly like any teenager, and stays in bed for hours if he gets the chance. We got used to the early start, it was just part of his pattern. The house was as safe as we could make it and we kept our door open so we could hear him, though nine times out of ten we would probably get up with him anyway. That didn't worry me nearly as much as keeping the night terrors at bay.

Even now Zoe and Matt are in different rooms but he will pop in to talk to her in the night or he will come in to us pull the curtains back in the middle of the night and describe the clouds and the moon. He will offer to count the stars for you, but at 2 or 3 in the morning you just wish that he would go to sleep.

Medication – pros and cons

Some ASD children just can't switch off. Matt sometimes takes a drug called Melatonin, a natural hormone supplement that has a role in sleep cycles. When it was originally prescribed we used it quite a lot to get him into the pattern of bed/sleep. Once we got the pattern established I withdrew it and now he only has it when he really needs it, which is when he simply can't switch off. Sometimes he is so wound up that he just can't get to sleep, and when he is in a phase of that he will sometimes say 'I really need to sleep', and then we give him a little Melatonin.

I haven't used drugs for any other areas of behaviour with Matt. I have seen Ritalin work with other children and I have seen times when it has really helped, but I have also seen cases where it has made the child really dopey and not with it and, personally, I wanted Matt to be as much himself as possible. But then, he is a relatively mild case, and I would never think that parents should rule this out as a possibility. It is very much down to the individuals. I have seen cases where a child just can't slow down and Ritalin has made them much better.

Food problems

It was very apparent from a young age that whereas the others would eat anything Matt wouldn't, and he didn't even want to try things. Foods he didn't like would make him gag. I didn't want him to end up with a food phobia, so from when he was about three I used to get him to help me cook and try, smell, feel, touch, taste everything while we were cooking, so that he knew all the way through what the food was going to be like. I used to let him sit on the worktop while I was preparing food and taste and play with anything. He would taste things that were safe to eat raw before they were cooked and then again after they had been cooked, so he was following the process right the way through. It meant that he could understand the food, rather than just being confronted with it at meal times.

When he helped me cook it he was so proud that he had helped, and dishing it up for Dad and his brothers made him really happy. It helped him a lot and got him over a lot of phobias. If you do the same with your ASD child, do take a picture of the meal that you have both prepared to add to your picture/word collection.

Eggs have been a real problem until quite recently. I showed Matt pictures of hens and eggs and things that you could cook with eggs to help him. They do have a slimy texture, which he hates, but he doesn't mind eating eggs in cakes and things because then the texture has changed. I got eggs into his diet by cooking them in other things. It is only very recently that he has been able to eat them on their own.

When we went to the supermarket he would pick things up and smell them because that is how he identifies food. He often doesn't remember even foods we have regularly. If you ask if he would like a beefburger, which he has had hundreds of times, he will ask what it looks like so that he can think what it is.

I think the cooking was one of my biggest turnarounds with him and I am sure that it stopped an awful lot of fads with his food. Now I put everything in front of him and he will eat around ninety percent of what is offered.

I did the same with drinks because of the different colours, which fascinate him. If I changed to a different colour of washing up liquid he would have to taste it to see if it was the same because it looked different; even bleach and household cleaners got the same treatment if I wasn't careful. You name it he would try it, even though I put things right away and then labelled them with a sick sign, meaning that they would make you sick if you tried them; he wasn't tasting things to be naughty, just in a spirit of enquiry.

Once the boys brought home tadpoles and he picked one up, looked at it smelled it and then, before we could stop him, he ate it. He said that it was a bit slimy. Then he kept doing it every time the tadpole changed shape because to him it was something different then. When supermarkets change the wrapper on something, as far as he is concerned it is a new thing and has to be investigated all over again.

When Matt was younger, every day was a new day for all the impressions that he got and each everyday thing that he saw was a new thing. He was always smelling and tasting things in the house and garden or at the shops, as a way of getting to know them. Now he will say something like 'you've changed the colour of the washing up liquid' rather than having to taste it. That is through me telling him not to do it.

- Get poor eaters to help you cook – they will lose their suspicion of food if they understand how it is put together and may find it more interesting if they have made it themselves.

Different textures may become more acceptable this way, too.

- I worked with an autistic child who had a food phobia. I boiled up a load of spaghetti and put it on my nose, my head, throwing it and having a great time with it so he saw me being completely unafraid of it and having fun with it so he wanted to join in and have fun and after that he was not afraid of touching it. Gradually you could broaden something like that out to other foods.
- Incidentally, almost all the children I have dealt with have had digestive problems where they find it really hard to go to the loo in a normal way. How can a child with no speech tell you they are constipated? A lot of their distressed behaviour could come down to a cause as simple as this. Do watch out for this if you can't see anything else that might be causing a behaviour problem.

Time keeping

Matt can tell the time but it doesn't mean much to him. If I tell him he needs to be in at a certain time he may try, but he is easily distracted if he bumps into someone or something happens. He does understand the concept of lateness now because every time he was late he found he wasn't allowed out the following night. When he loses something he wants to do, it does register. I would tell him that if he was on time he could go out again the following night. We worked on this for ages and even now I still do it because you have to keep up the continuity. Unfortunately, we find that if Matt has asked once if he can go out he forgets to ask again if he can go somewhere else at a different time. I couldn't say that Matt has ever really grasped the concept of being on time, but anyway here are some things that we have found helped a bit and could help you.

- Give your child a watch.
- Write the time you need him to be back on his hand.
- Let him have a mobile phone and make sure it is switched on.
- Try using a timer that goes off in his pocket.

These are all useful things to try. Matt still switches off the phone or timer then forgets that he is supposed to be somewhere or meeting someone.

Being quick

ASD children can't rush, and you can't make them rush, because, if you do that, you are asking them to do too many things in one go: to think of the time, to get ready, to think about getting out of the door, all at once. And they will be very easily distracted.

- Egg timer – give a reward if the child beats the egg timer.
- Have a reward ready to give in the car if your child has been quick.

Remembering

Matt has a total lack of short-term memory. He can have

something in his hand and I will say 'go and put this in your school bag in the next room' and he will forget before he gets there. He has no sense of urgency, he just can't entertain the concept of hurrying or being on time, so getting to school each morning can be a real problem.

- To help them remember what they need for the day try making a laminated checklist (either using words or pictures) of items they need for school. Punch a hole in it and put it on a chain attached to their school bag. 'Have I got homework/ reading book/sports kit/lunch box/coat?' With a list like this they can check for themselves and feel in control.

Dressing

Here you will encounter the difficulties of an extremely literal approach to instructions – they will do **exactly** what you say, so you have to say **exactl**y what you want them to do. I have always reminded Matt what clothes to put on in the morning and in what order. When I walk past his room I give the whole sequence of dressing instructions one thing at a time – right down to each sock and each shoe. Very gradually that has improved. Once, when his father was getting him ready for school, he ended up setting off without his shoes because nobody had reminded him to put them on.

- Make a picture wall chart of the clothes he puts on in the morning and a timetable of his routine – e.g. wash/dress/ breakfast and put it next to a clock on the wall to help with timing as well (if you are lucky!)

Out and about

You can give an instruction to an autistic child, they can parrot it back to you but they don't know what it means so they can't put it into practice. For instance, I taught Matt the Green Cross Code so he knew the words that told him that he had to stand at the kerb, but when I took him out into the road he couldn't relate the rhyme in his head to what he actually had to do. Saying the Green Cross Code aloud as you are doing it can help, but I found crossing the road the same way every time more help as it became routine. Matt would just go off if he saw something interesting, so I got a wrist-to-wrist attachment and used it for ages, and when he was too old for that he **had** to hold someone's hand when he was out or he would be off.

- If you have a real wanderer get a tracking device or one of those key rings that bleep and attach it to their clothes when you go out so that you can find them and they know that you can find them.

Travelling in the car

Another thing Matt did, which it took me a long time to understand, was that if we travelled somewhere he would suddenly start screaming and trying to get himself out of his seatbelt, while the others were trying to hold him in. He would be screaming that he needed England, sweating with nerves and flapping his arms. Once we were on the dual carriageway and he tried to open the door to get out. At that point we had to change the car to one with no doors at the back that he could open. He knew that England was where he lived and where home was, but if I took a different route to normal he thought that he was leaving England and losing everything familiar. He didn't like it if you changed routes or routines, because he always wanted everything to be the same. I had to spend a lot of time with him using a map to show him that the route would bring us back and I showed him that the road on the map was called Wisteria Avenue and we were parked in Wisteria Avenue, so he could relate the map to what we were doing Then he started saying things like 'this is just a different road isn't it – we are going to the same place but just on a different road.'

- Photocopy a map and draw the road you take so the child can follow it and not get anxious. The next time you do that journey take a slightly different route with a different marking on the map. He can see it all ends up in the same place so he can get used to changing routes and spare you all from some agitation.

If I took Matt into a multi-storey car park at this time he would just go berserk because there were cars pulling in, pulling out, going one way, going the other way and he couldn't keep his eyes on what was going on around him. He is still quite afraid of traffic, though now he can cope. I actually took him into car parks and sat in the car with him for a long time when he was little and let him watch the cars. It helped when I explained that if there was an arrow on the floor they had to go that way. Once he knew there was a structure and rules he turned a corner on that particular anxiety. Now we can go into multi-storey car parks without him getting upset. Often he will remark on how many cars there are there, but he has learned to cope with the anxiety of what is going on around him

Shopping

Have a list of foods you need and let them help look for them; this also helps with memory and recognition and helps you to get your shopping done more quickly. If your child does not like shopping, ask someone to look after them while you do the shopping; remember people with ASD generally do not like places where there are a lot of people. Again you are respecting them for who they are. You can get over this fear by slowly getting them to help you do the shopping, by going to small shops first and working your way up to big stores.

- Have a list. It is quicker and will keep them occupied.
- Explain to them why people do not like it when you smell food in shops, and go over this lots of times.
- Show them that no one else in the shop is doing this.
- Explain that you can leave the shop more quickly if they help.
- Most of all, reward them at the end of the shopping trip, perhaps by buying something they like to collect, such as a magazine or stickers or a treat such as something to eat.

Holidays

We always go to the same place on holiday – the one time we went somewhere different it took Matt such ages to relax that none of us could really wind down.

- You can prepare them for a holiday by using a map to show them the route you are going to use.
- Tell them all about what to expect when they get there.
- Take some familiar things with you to make them feel at home.

Chapter 10

Getting organised can save your sanity

You need to be very organized as a parent of an ASD child, especially when there are other children in the family, too. I have found if you are disorganized the household becomes very stressful to all and anxiety is not just the child's problem but yours too!

To avoid this, look at all you do and make it your job to get it right. If you have an aim and purpose you will find it easier; I know I do.

How to modify your home

Just look around and you will find lots of simple things you can do in your house that will make everyone's lives run more smoothly.

- Although a child with ASD is often pretty noisy, they can also be sensitive to noise. You can reduce noise levels in your house with carpets instead of wood or laminate flooring.
- Soft lighting is kinder than harsh fluorescent light.
- It can be helpful to ASD children if the furniture is around

the edges of the room, with the middle space kept fairly clear.

- Patterns can be confusing and anxiety-inducing to walk or sit on, so keep carpets and furnishings as plain as you can.
- Duvets, bean bags and comfy chairs can help ASD children feel safer and more calm.
- Make sure your house is as safe as it can be. Foil escape artists wherever possible. ASD children have little sense of danger, so prepare for the unexpected. Have locks for windows and cupboards, and keep plug covers in use long term. An ASD child really never grows out of tinkering with things.
- One idea is to put bells on all your doors, with different chimes for different doors, so you know which room your child is going into and can keep track of them around the house – or if they are trying to get out of the house.
- After the distressing incident when Matt cleaned his teeth with haemorrhoid cream instead of toothpaste, I locked all the medical stuff in a box on a high shelf in the bathroom that he couldn't reach, and we have kept it there ever since.
- Try to give them their own space to chill out and calm down when they need to. They need this as much as anyone else does, probably more.
- Somewhere to exercise and let off steam is brilliant. For instance, trampolines are often a great success.
- Check that you don't have anything poisonous in the house, and that includes plants.

- Pictures of objects to help the child understand what they have to do, such as get dressed in the morning, get ready for school, can be stuck in appropriate places around the house.

Think of it as your JOB. OK, it's unpaid, but well worth it. You are your own boss so you can make your own timetable of the day, one that works for you and the rest of the family. Keep to your timetable it will help you and your family to get organized.

Be prepared for things to go wrong and work out how to deal with them if they do, so you can stay on track.

How to modify your life

- Make packed lunches the night before and make all your children pack their school bags the night before; make a timetable that takes problems into account.
- Be generous with your timing so you don't need to rush. If something goes wrong you have time to spare so you won't have to get tense and worried about being late.
- Don't set your targets too high to start with. If you fail at something you will feel bad about it and that is no good for you.
- If you want to go out in the morning get things ready the night before. You can even pack the car up, then you don't have to rush.
- Lay the clothes out the night before ready for your ASD

child to put on in the morning; ask what they would like to wear to wherever you are going.

I use printed timetables to help me keep track of my observations with Matt and I find them really useful, so I have put in a couple as examples. You can ask for this to be done in school as well, which can help to pinpoint any daily difficulties, and helps with liaison between home and school.

HOME

Date	Time	Target	Comment
10/7/05	7am	Get up	Still finds this hard need to wake him slowly
10/7/05	7.15am	Have a wash	Remember to say each item: flannel, soap, wash face, etc;
10/7/05	7.30am	Get dressed	Needs help with buttons, need to practise more
10/7/0/5	7.45am	Have breakfast	Eat with a spoon, still need to practise
10/7/05	8.00am	Get in car	Needs more time

The timetable shows me that I need more time to help Matt get out in the morning so I need to wake the whole family up earlier.

SCHOOL

Date	Time	Target	Comment
10/7/05	9.00am	Sit in registration	Sat for 3 mins need to work on sitting use egg timer
10/7/05	9.15 am.	Do 4 sums in maths, then practical maths	Found this hard today, got 2 sums done then did practical maths next time I will go back to the last 2 sums
10/7/05	9.45 am	Go over writing in English lesson	Find hand eye co-ordination hard
10/7/05	10.15am	Break time – try to sit and eat fruit with other children	Does not like to sit and eat with other children so I sat with him and encouraged him – keep it going

As you can see it is very straightforward. It helps a lot as, if your child gets cross, it is all logged. This helps as a way to keep track of what progress your child is making at home or school

Chapter 11

Schooling

Mainstream versus special schools

Deciding what kind of education is going to be best for your ASD child is one of the hardest decisions that you are going to have to make. There is a lot to be said in favour of both mainstream and special schooling, although in some areas lack of a decent choice means that the decision is virtually made for you. Parents faced with the dilemma of deciding what is best for their child often don't know all their rights in this area, and they may face a real battle.

Government policy is veering towards special needs inclusion in mainstream education wherever possible, so special schools provision is very limited in some areas and mainstream teachers need more specialised training and acceptance of their role. There is a need for more specialist attention in mainstream schools where some teachers still have scant understanding of the problems ASD children face.

Within the framework of what is available, the most important thing when you are making a decision is to base it on the character of your child and what is likely to be best for him or her. A child's intelligence level is nothing to do with whether they are within the spectrum or not, so your decision will not be made purely on academic grounds. Make a list of their needs and consider how each one will be met, and also make a list of the important features of each way of educating and how they match up with your child's needs. For instance, sending a nervous, clingy child away to boarding school would probably be torture for you both, however good the facilities, although for a different type of child it might offer possibilities of independence that would be entirely beneficial.

Mainstream school – our choice for Matt and how we made it

We chose to send Matt to the same local school that his brothers had attended. I wanted him to follow the lead of ordinary children and I felt that it was important for him to develop his social skills. That did influence my decision to go for mainstream school.

I didn't think Matt was independent enough to go away from home to special school, as a boarding school was the only option available to us, and I also felt that as a parent I would be letting him down if I sent him away. I didn't want someone else to take over things I felt I should be doing myself.

If there had been a special day school that could have offered Matt what he needed, my decision might have changed. Some children might well be happier in an environment where they do not feel so different, such as a special school where everyone is like them. I felt that it would cut down on Matt's chances to assimilate into the real world and to experience life, even if he is led a bit of a dance by some of his friends at mainstream school and maybe gets to experience a bit too much sometimes.

One negative aspect of mainstream schooling is that not all the teachers understand or appreciate the difficulties of an ASD child. I think the parent/teacher relationship is difficult with special needs. You have to be able to feel sure that they want the best for your child and there needs to be considerable understanding and support on both sides. As a special needs learning support assistant who is also a parent of an ASD child I hope I have more compassion than is often the case.

As a parent you have to let the teachers do their job, although that can be hard. One thing you can do is give the teachers a folder with all the relevant information on how you talk to and discipline your child, things that you feel would be helpful when they are dealing with him.

With the policy of inclusion in primary schools there is far more chance for children to assimilate differences without really being aware. Having a physical disability is easier for them to see and understand than a disability like Matt's, where people can look and talk normally but then behave inappropriately. Children pick it up much quicker than adults, but some handle it better than others. I want Matt to be himself and to do that everyone has to accept him for who he is; when he does something that seems odd, that is part of Matt.

Of course there are lots of other educational choices to bear in mind, and I thought the best way of looking at them was to talk to people involved in different areas to find out the good – and the bad – points that might help you with a decision.

The compromise solution – introducing special needs into the mainstream

Zena Fisher, Matt's respite carer works at a special school, which has an innovative approach to inclusion.'I work as inclusion facilitator at a special school so I take children with special needs from the special school into the mainstream, as part of a new scheme piloted by the local education authority. I feel that if you can include as much as possible for each individual child then that is the ideal.

'Children who go to the special school get specialist input from experienced and knowledgeable teachers; they can have hydrotherapy, speech therapy and physiotherapy if they need it, and they can go in and out of mainstream school for the subjects they can manage or even just for social inclusion. I take 26 children from our school to a mainstream primary for different sessions according to their needs. That includes two severely autistic children with no verbal communication but who are absolutely brilliant on computers. They go in to year 9 computer lessons and they are very skilled, although they could never tell you how they did it. They need stretching in that area which they would not get at the special school. Another autistic child I take is fantastic at art so he goes in and you can tell that he really enjoys his lessons, although socially he doesn't care where he is.

'This way these children have the best of both worlds. They really benefit from the stimulation at the mainstream school and, at the same time, being at the top of the group at special school does wonders for their self-esteem, whereas, if they were full time in mainstream, they might sink without a trace.'

Special school – when state provision really works

There is enormous pressure on special school places in most parts of the country, so Lesley Burton feels that she was very lucky to get a place at a local state special school for her son, Eddie. 'Because we got our diagnosis early we were advised to get Eddie a place at a school which is not too far from home and gives him the autism specific provision he needs. But the bureaucratic procedure of getting assessments, a statement of Special Educational Needs (in order to qualify for a place) is quite laborious. I hounded the Education authority to ensure Eddie's case was heard at the first opportunity and all the correct documents had been submitted to the right people. However, we felt it was worth it. Eddie was given a place, is very happy at this school and has really made progress. There are not nearly enough places at his school or at similar schools around the country and people are just crying out for them. The school uses a mix of TEACCH and some ABA methods. Eddie is not verbal and uses PECS to communicate. He started at the school at age three and could stay until he is 18. In just over a year it has made such a difference to my little boy, to his behaviour and cognitive ability – he is learning, he is alert, he is interacting more. The whole programme is geared to communication. They have interaction the whole time, which not all schools offer, so the children are not just dealing with adults on a one-to-one basis but with children of their own age, albeit all with difficulties. They say that, surprisingly for an autistic child, Eddie does seek out play with the other children, perhaps because he has a brother and sister at home. Because he wants someone else to be on the seesaw, someone else to throw the ball to, he will initiate contact, which is fantastic, and we are encouraged by his current progress and happiness at school to think that he is really in the right place for now. Ironically, if, after all this help, he is considered to be at the 'high functioning' end of the autistic spectrum, the provision here is non-existent, which will throw up a whole new set of problems.'

Special needs units within mainstream schools – winners in the postcode lottery

Alexander Lubbock is 12 and is a pupil at a Chinnor Unit, within a state school. These are self-contained units in several Oxfordshire schools, which allow pupils to integrate into main school classes where it is beneficial. His father, John Lubbock is pleased with the merits of this type of structure. 'You can go right through school as an autistic child in the system. The unit is brilliant, completely self-contained and almost one to one staff, but they can go out into the school for whatever they can manage. Some don't go at all, some go a lot. Alexander is a very clever boy but he is quite severely autistic. It is better for him to be out in the world than not. He does PE in the main school and he does drama and he has a tutor group, which is a pastoral thing. He also joins them for lunch and play. He doesn't socialise at all, he pretty much ignores everybody, but he is happy that he is there and he is proud that he is in a proper school with ordinary people and he is capable of dealing with it all.

Within the special unit he does things that are specifically geared up to his needs. They go on outings together and go to the shops and go swimming and some participate more than others. He tends to get pretty involved but then when they are in the unit at their own desk it is pretty much geared to each child. The primary school was a Chinnor unit as well, we are very lucky to live in Oxfordshire. He went into the special unit every week for a year from his primary school, which was an excellent way to prepare him for the change, but he was very shocked when he realised that his primary school teacher would not be coming with him. He found it very hard to settle in, but they did help him.'

The academic mainstream – problems for a high achieving Asperger's sufferer

Finni Golden's son, Jamie, is highly academic, but as someone with mild Asperger's, life at school has had its problems for him. 'Jamie has the normal problems associated with Asperger's in his social life, but not particularly in his educational life. He is very intelligent – he understands concepts and is very clear thinking. He lives in a very philosophical household so there is not much chance of him not getting involved in various debates. He is clever, conscientious and hard working but he is driven by a terrible perfectionism and he suffers terribly with OCDs, which are his nightmare. Part of that has a good result in that he likes to get everything finished and it has to be done perfectly, so I don't have to stand over him with a stick to get homework done. As with a lot of these conditions you do have to find and respect the positive.

'A special school would probably never have been a suitable option for him but mainstream school is particularly difficult for children like him who are generally not good at any sport because they often have motor problems with co-ordination and so on. Jamie gets teased for being an egghead and a nerd and all those awful things that children taunt each other with. He is quite hot headed as well, which I think goes with the general anger at being different, so he will retaliate to his own detriment.

'It took me a long time to realise that it really takes him about four years to settle in to a school. When I felt he was unhappy at his first school I decided to move him, but by the time I had researched new schools, got him through the entrance exams and moved house to be near his new prep school, he had really settled into the school where he had been so unhappy and I realised that he does need a lot of time to adjust. The best advice I could give to someone in a similar situation is persevere where you are if you can, because it doesn't actually matter which school you put them in, they are initially going to have a very difficult time with some of the other children. Jamie has always had problems in that he is probably three years younger than his age socially and three years older academically. He learned to read when he was two and was keen to know about everything. He demanded to know what letters and symbols meant almost before he could speak.

'At prep school he found it very hard before the diagnosis of Asperger's and I just thought I had a very bright and difficult child. It didn't help that diagnosis of Asperger's didn't come until he was $9^1/_2$, by which time he had got into the Grammar School, where he goes now.

'For me personally things have got easier now I understand the difficulties and have the patience to realise that if I spend ages teaching him to tie up the laces on his gym shoes I will have to spend the same amount of time teaching him to tie up the laces on his school shoes because they are different shoes. There is no blueprint so everything has to be learned for the first time. In his world there are no received ideas at all. Once you have learned the patience involved with coping with that it is not a problem.

'His teachers are generally sympathetic, but whether they have done anything positive to help him is another matter. It has been easier for him as he has got older because, in education generally, they are very much more aware of the problems these days and they have things in place. Having originally known nothing about Jamie's condition, six years on the school has a system in place with a specific member of staff to help with special learning difficulties.

'At the gifted end of the spectrum, mainstream education is something my son has coped with, but it has not been easy by any stretch of the imagination. Academically able children have a different set of problems. They need to be stretched by their education, otherwise it is very frustrating for someone clever. I still regret that I didn't know his diagnosis right from the outset because then I would definitely have sent him to a Steiner school where they seem to educate the whole person, not just the brain.'

Home education

Although home education is sometimes a first choice, it is often a response to problems with mainstream education. This was certainly the case for Elaine Holyer, who felt very strongly that her son James was at a school that was unable to meet his special needs. 'After years of battling to get a statement and then battling to get the school to keep to the provisions of it – after all it is a document of law – I felt very let down by the system. I was told that our area is known not to be a good provider of special needs education, but that is really no comfort at all.

'I am very pleased with our decision to home educate. I don't think that James had really learned anything in his two years at secondary school. Help was just not geared towards him. I had to fight to get him a teaching assistant and, as she was previously a lollipop lady, and was taken on without any training, nice as she was, she couldn't really help with his work. James had not really learned any decent maths since year one, when he was five, and he is now 13, so with some initial help from a friend who is a teacher, I have started on a programme which aims to give him a proper working familiarity with numbers. As we have gone on, it has become clear that his brain hasn't been used much in that area, so we do a lot of mental maths. One of the advantages of home educating is that you really can gear things to the specific needs of your child, which in our case are compounded by the fact that James has Pathological Demand Avoidance Syndrome, as well as Asperger's. He will comply only if you approach things in the right way, and I have come up with my own methods of dealing with him, which are far more effective than for him to be just sitting in a classroom doing nothing.

'There seem to be no set rules on home education, but I have had some useful guidelines on my rights from the organisation Education Otherwise.

'**www.education-otherwise.org** (helpline 0870-7300074) also organises various group outings and activities for members, thus ensuring some level of social contact.

'Also, **www.he-special.org.uk** has resources for home educating a child with special educational needs.'

Prospective home educators often worry about issues of social integration that can be crucial for ASD children. Those who have taken the plunge tend to be adamant that their children do not miss out socially. Certainly, you can make sure that there are plenty of out-of-school activities, sports and clubs to fill in the social gaps, but it does seem that an element of isolation is built in to this choice, and if you feel that your child needs the regular company of other children to learn essential social skills (even if they might actually be happier in solitary state) then you need to consider this option carefully.

Things to consider when you make your choice

MAINSTREAM SCHOOL

- Will give a chance to integrate more into the everyday world.
- May be the best option for academically able children.
- May require ASD children to conform to rules that baffle them and punish for non-compliance.
- May not have special needs qualified teachers – quite unlikely to have had an opportunity to do any courses on autism.
- Teachers may not understand your child's problems.
- Teachers calling you in for every little thing your child does making you feel awful and not understanding your problems at all.
- Not all mainstream schools have the capability to address complex needs.
- ASD children are very vulnerable to bullying and can be miserable in the mainstream.

SPECIAL SCHOOL

- Will understand your child and his or her ways.
- More hands on teaching, more one to one.
- Will give the chance to be with others like them – this may not be such a good thing for those with ASD.

- May not push your child enough – there can be a tendency to settle at the lowest common denominator.
- Teachers with specialist skills are more likely to be found in special schools.
- Small groups/work geared to their ability/lots of support/good for confidence.
- Children used to a small group may well become anxious and unable to function properly in a big mainstream class. This often becomes an issue on transfer from primary to secondary.
- ASD children get a feeling of security and routine from a small special school.

The main point is that for some children the stimulus of the mainstream is important, while for others the sheltered environment of a special school may give them the security they need. The choice should be available to all, so that each individual child can benefit from the education that best suits him. Sadly, at present, this choice is seldom available to ASD children and their parents.

You have to look at what is best for the individual child. Matt, for instance, would not have coped in a special school. I wanted him to have normal experiences and in consequence we have had problems with him trying smoking, skiving off school and all the rest. Clearly, this would not be the right solution for everyone; some children simply couldn't survive the mainstream. People who understand ASD will know that children like Matt are often happier at school than at home, because you don't have rigid timetables at home and you do at school – and of course they find that very reassuring.

Useful contacts

- The Advisory Centre for Education (ACE) is an independent charity offering information about state education and telephone advice on subjects such as special educational needs. **www.ace-ed.org.uk** (helpline 0808 8005793).
- Network 81 – a national network of parents working towards properly resourced inclusive education for children with special needs (helpline 0870 770 3306).
- Parents for Inclusion is a national charity set up with the aim of helping disabled children learn, make friends and have a voice in ordinary school **www.parentsforinclusion.org** (helpline 0800 652 3145).

Chapter 12

Problems at school

Some schools really don't want to deal with ASD children because it means they have to put themselves out to teach them, but in the current climate where inclusion when possible is the stated aim, they have to move with the times.

In meetings with Matt's school I know I have sometimes found it really hard not to yell out 'but that is your job, to accommodate each child's needs'. The thing is that there is a knack to teaching autistic children. You do have to deal with them in a different way to the rest of the class and I know it is hard. I make mistakes myself and I live with the problem every day, so I know it is hard for outsiders. Schools should try to understand what a struggle it can be for special needs parents, and be more sympathetic. A recent report said that nearly half of parents in the category experienced problems with the educational system, and I can well believe it.

So, given that the system imposes strains both on parent and teacher – not to mention the pupil – what can you do as a parent to make things easier for everyone? One thing is to promote awareness of what your child's condition, in our case Asperger's syndrome, will mean for the teacher.

It helps if the teacher knows that:

- ASD children will find it really hard to learn the social skills they need for school, and may not have many reserves left for class work – at least initially. Such children may also find it hard to understand the need to fit in and obey the rules.
- A teacher needs to be very explicit in giving instructions and check that the child has really understood them and knows what they are meant to do. The teacher should start instructions with the child's name or he may not realise that he is the one being talked to.
- It will help if the teacher bears in mind that this child may not understand visual clues from facial expression or behaviour or have much idea of the effect of his behaviour on other children.
- A child with ASD will prefer familiar things and may resist moving from what he knows.
- The teacher may feel that the point of a lesson is obvious, but the ASD child may focus on something quite different.

These are just a few of the basic issues that the teacher is going to have to take on board when your child enters the class. There are guidelines available, but it will help everyone if you bear in mind that the teacher is having to make a lot of effort to incorporate your child's needs into what may well be a full and lively class, and be understanding in your approach as a parent.

I think more practical training and understanding of how ASD children function would be a huge help and I don't think that there is enough of it anywhere. I think the learning support assistants (LSAs – in class to give one-to-one support for each child with special needs) who work with these children need to be chosen very carefully and properly trained so that they understand the ASD child's condition and needs. An LSA is a crucial element in mainstream education for boys like Matthew, but LSA training for special needs, which is not compulsory anyway, does not go into certain conditions, including ASD. So the people directly involved in their day-to-day school life may not have any specific training. Even one week's specific training would make everybody's life so much easier.

If you get the chance to talk things through with your LSA, you can make sure that they understand what they will be dealing with.

The LSA needs to know how to:

- Interpret situations for the child and show them what they need to do, using simple language and one instruction at a time and always going at the child's pace.
- Help them learn social skills such as turn taking, while guiding other children in the class in how to interact with them.
- Understand an ASD child's problems with language and communication and make things clear to them when they are confused.
- Anticipate and try to avoid things that will cause anxiety.
- Appreciate that the approach for an ASD child is different

to other special needs. They may be happy with the routine and structure of fairly solitary learning and uncomfortable with playing with classmates.

School life by Matthew Keith Brealy

'When i wake up i find it hard because my body feels like staying in bed. Once i do get up and have to put my clothes on ,sometimes i forget to put my boxers on and just put my trousers on. when i have to pack my bag i need to rember to pack my .pe. kit because all the time i forget. sometimes i have not rembered to clean my teeth and little things like that. when i get to school i go to my first lesson. the teacher dosent give me enough time to get my stuff ready. when they ask a question they don't give me enough time to answer them. your brain needs to think so then they asked someone else and i get a low mark and i get funny spells if i get them when a teacher is speaking to me i have to make them say it again and they get annoyed with me.if a teacher shouts at me i laugh because i find it funny .i prefer if they talk to me and not shout at me . i don't like it when a teacher has shouted at me because i did something wrong and i don't reliase what i've done.'

How to make schooldays less stressful.

Sad to say, parents in mainstream school can probably expect hostility from other parents who feel that ASD children are just disruptive and hog the teacher's time and attention. This is something that you need to be prepared for. I feel there should be more liaison with other parents and teachers for ASD parents, maybe mediation from someone like myself who understands both sides of the situation at first hand. If the school is not being helpful or understanding, what can you do?

How can you sort out continuing problems with a particular teacher?

- You need to keep in touch with your child's work and progress so you know and understand what the teacher is saying.
- If the teacher is hard to talk to, go to the special needs teacher and explain your worries. He or she should be able to help you.
- You should take on board what the teacher has to say as you need to be able to see the situation from both sides.
- If you are still unhappy with the results you need to see the head and ask for an action plan to be made to help all concerned.
- You can go to the educational psychologist for the school area who will help put an individual education plan together which can help everyone who is concerned with the child.
- If all else fails, you can ask that your child is not taught by this teacher but it is best if you can meet half way.
- Teachers don't always realise that they have to explain things over and over again to ASD children, so if you can – tactfully – remind them of the parameters of the condition; it will help

Trouble in class by Matthew Keith Brealy

'I've lost count of how many times I've been in trouble because the teacher has told me to copy a question from the board. I do it, because that's what

I've been asked to do, but then I get in trouble for not putting the answer down too. But he didn't ask me to do that.'

It doesn't matter how often this happens, Matt still won't realise – so the teacher should. Children like Matt will only do what they are asked. He gets put outside the classroom door for not concentrating. When the teacher asks Matt if he will come back in now and concentrate he will say 'no', because he knows he can't concentrate, and then his reply gets him into even more trouble. This still happens routinely, and he is 14 now.

Of course, Matt is not an entirely innocent victim in all this. Whenever the teacher gets cross at school, Matt gleefully watches her face go red. To him it is funny that the redness starts at her chin and goes all the way up her face. He notices things like that which others might not even register, he wants to get a reaction from her so that he can see that red face. People think that Matt's attitude is confrontational because if an LSA says that he needs to do something he will always say 'why?' I am sure that that is really irritating, but, unfortunately, he really does want to know why.

Matt is always losing his pencil case and other stuff and he gets punished. He will take it out of his bag to put something in and then forget to put it back. Then he gets frustrated and surprised because he knows he started the day off with it and is baffled by its disappearance. His problems in school, I'm afraid, are fairly typical. It is a widespread problem. The National Autistic Society says that over 10 per cent of queries it receives each year are education related.

I started training in special needs when my daughter started school and I saw a girl there who was just like Matt. I helped out with her and then did an NVQ. I found that I really enjoyed the studying and had learned so much from Matt, which I took into my special needs teaching. What pushed me into it was that Matt was having so many problems at school and I wondered how many other parents were having the same problems.

Matt does hands-on subjects at school. He has the concentration of a gnat, he is so easily distracted and has little memory, then he gets in trouble because he can't remember. I would have liked him to repeat a year but the special needs teacher felt that it was important for Matt to be quite cool and in with his mates and it would be humiliating for him to be kept down with younger ones. School is more important socially and for the acquisition of life skills than it is academically for him. It is not worth him pushing for exams and we will look in the direction of practical jobs when he finishes.

There are still a handful of parents who don't want their children to play with anyone not 'normal' and so the cycle of prejudice continues. I think it is good that they have to be more inclusive in schools. I think it may make other parents confront their prejudices a bit.

Those difficult times of day

ASSEMBLY

Assembly has all the ingredients an ASD child will hate: noisy groups going into and out of the hall, the necessity to sit quietly, in closely packed rows, where they may be stuck in the middle rather than at the edges which they would prefer, and then the need to sit quiet and still while someone goes on and on about something boring. There are lots of rules here that are different to the classroom and may be hard to grasp. If you think your child is going to have trouble with all this when they start school there are a few things you could try.

- Ask if he has to go into assembly right from the start, especially if you think it will make him anxious. Maybe he could spend some quiet time with a one-to-one activity before the hustle of the day in class.
- If he can gradually start coming into assembly at his own pace, success may be more likely.
- Make sure he understands the rules and what he has to do, and see if there is another child who can help him out and keep an eye on him and be his 'buddy'. If he has a one-to-one helper they should sit with him.
- Ask if he can sit at the edge so that he will feel more comfortable.
- Explain how long Assembly will last – use egg timers to help with the idea of the time.

BREAK TIME

Break time is quite often hard for ASD children as it is not structured. When they are uncertain what to do they may act inappropriately or isolate themselves from other children, so you may need to ask someone to organise their play. Matt usually hangs around with his friends and sometimes gets into trouble, which I feel is all a learning point. Here are some things you can try to help with break times:

- Encourage them to join a break time club.
- Ask to see if they can sit in the library.
- See if the school uses the 'buddy' system, which is where another child is your child's special companion and helps them play or sits and reads with them.
- If your child likes to be alone then find out if there is a suitable place for them.
- See if the school has a time out room (where children can go to be on their own and undisturbed).
- If they want to join in with the others, but don't know how, try to teach them some ways to start up conversations without people thinking they are weird.

LUNCH TIME

Lunch is a noisy and sociable time that can be a nightmare for an ASD child, who will need strategies to help them to cope.

- Try to get their teacher or support assistant to role play the lunchtime routine when the dining room is empty and quiet.
- If they find queuing difficult see if the teachers will let them be at the front or back of the queue, rather than anywhere in the middle, which may make them very anxious.

- Make sure the dinner ladies know what has been arranged for them.
- Try to teach them a few simple bits of conversation to help them to join in with the children at their table.

Working with classmates

Joining in with others can be very problematical for your ASD child, who may not have much awareness of the feelings of other people or of the effect his or her behaviour can have on them. Some ASD children will be tense and anxious if someone is even sitting too near them. Working in groups is the norm for a lot of lessons these days, so you will need some strategies to help your child get used to working with others.

- You know how much social contact your child can cope with before anxiety sets in: make sure the teacher knows too.
- Ask if your child can sit at the edge of group activity to start with, perhaps on the other side of the support assistant.
- The support assistant can encourage your child to try turn-taking tasks, at first with him or her and then in a supervised way with another child, then, if all goes well, just with the other child.
- Tell the teacher of any special skills or interests your child has which she may be able to draw on in class.
- If your child can cope with it invite a classmate to your house for tea. It can be very helpful if you encourage this before your child starts at the school.

Staying in school

Matt has a bad habit of wandering off site during the day. If he wants to buy a drink or something, he will just go to the shop, quite forgetting that he is supposed to stay in the school grounds. Now I have put a laminated note in his bag where his money is which reads 'Matt don't leave the school premises' and that seems to do the trick.

School holidays

Most ASD children find the disruption to routine of the school holidays rather a hard thing to cope with. Matt used to be awful, but now he loves the holidays best. I found that starting up a timetable at home has sorted out the problem.

- Timetable each day of the holidays.
- Work out what you are going to do and keep it structured.
- Get your child to help with the timetable.
- Let them help choose activities.
- Have a time out zone in the house in case things get too much. If there is one at school your child will probably want one at home, too.

Other problems

BULLYING

This is a worry for all parents, and children with any disability can be especially vulnerable to bullying. I was lucky as Matt's older brother was at the same school and he took good care of him, but you still get the odd day where other children do say things that upset your child. On the other hand, children with ASD can say the most awful things to other children, and I have used this fact to explain to Matt how people feel when he says mean things to them. With other ASD children I have worked on making up a 'feelings folder' with different pictures showing feelings like sad / happy /cross; then asking them how they are feeling themselves and how they think what they have said has made someone else feel. The child will point to the picture and you can explain the feeling to them as best you can. As we know, ASD children tend to have real problems with relating to others socially; misunderstanding and lack of eye contact mean that they have immense difficulty interpreting much communication.

HOW TO HELP COMBAT BULLYING

- 'Buddy' them with someone at school – an older child or more mature classmate.
- Help them understand bullying – from both sides.
- Let them read the bullying leaflets.
- Listen to your child and watch out for unaccountable changes in behaviour, so you can see the special needs teacher as soon as any bullying starts.
- Keep a diary on your child – a pattern behind the bullying might emerge.
- For a child without speech you need an illustrated 'feelings folder' so they can show you what is wrong.

- Think of your child's feelings but also think that your child might be the one who is provoking the bullying by saying unkind things.

USEFUL CONTACTS

Advisory Centre for Education (ACE) **www.ace-ed.org.uk** (helpline 0808 8005793) offers telephone advice on bullying

Bullying Online **www.bullying.co.uk**

Some ways to make school life run more smoothly for your ASD child

- Allow plenty of time to get ready in the morning. If the child is rushed to start with, they will be anxious all day and will not concentrate.
- Make sure the child has packed up everything they need for that day.
- If you have other children, enlist their help as much as possible so that you can concentrate on helping your ASD child to get ready.
- Make sure you drop off at the same time and place each day.
- Picking them up at the same time, same place each night also helps routine.
- Have a drink and a snack ready when you pick them up after school to help them unwind.
- Give them the space and quiet time they need to unwind after school.

- Give the teacher written information to help get to know your child. I prepared a detailed folder on Matt, his ways and how we deal with him at home.
- If something has happened which has made the child anxious – a favourite toy has gone missing, their shirt is the Wrong One, or any one of countless other daily catastrophes – you need to tell the teacher first thing or they cannot make allowances for any change in behaviour and this will upset everyone.

Chapter 13

Know your rights

STATEMENTING

What is a statement and why do you need one?

If your child has been diagnosed with ASD then it is in your interests to secure a Statement of Special Educational Needs. The Statement is a legal document which sets out your child's needs and the help they should have, as determined by a local education authority assessment. This assessment aims to establish what your child's special educational needs are and comprises reports from the parent, the child's teacher, an educational psychologist, a paediatrician or doctor, and any others who are already helping your child. It is reviewed annually, with the stated aim of ensuring that the support given continues to meet the needs of your child.

A statement is vital if you wish to get any special provision for your child, such as special schooling, a learning support assistant in a mainstream class, speech therapy and much more besides. The advantages are that it is useful for the school to know what level of extra help they need to give. Matt has one to one help in the classroom and for changing and other things he needs.

Problems with getting a statement

I have two bulging files at home full of the correspondence it took to get Matt statemented. I really wanted to have his needs acknowledged and helped – and in order to do that I had to have a statement of special educational needs. There were times during the lengthy and tortuous process when I felt as if everyone was against me. A lot of people have the same experience and I really wonder why it has to be so hard and why you always feel as if you are in combat with the system.

I wish I had pushed things and got Matt statemented earlier. This was a huge battle as the school Matt was in said he was not bad enough to get a statement and they would not do it, but most days Matt came home from school with a problem or would run out of school and come home.

After I had Matt's diagnosis in hand and went to the school to show the head that Matt needed help he said in a very nasty way 'Well if Matthew has Asperger's syndrome then I have a school full.' He made it quite clear that he thought Matt was just naughty. I was shocked and very upset at being spoken to in this way. I left the school feeling really hurt. I had to find out where I stood on this. I knew the head teacher was not going to help me.

I was lucky really as I went to the library to find a book and on the notice board was a poster for a course called *Parents' guide to special needs statementing*. As you can imagine, I signed up straight away. The very fact that there are such courses is an indication of how often people need help with all this.

When I went to the first meeting I was so happy to find I was not the only parent struggling with hostile schools. I found out later that the reluctance to statement is often because of the cost, but what cost do you put on a child?

I did the eight-week course and found it well worth doing. I discovered that I could ask for a statement for my child without the school's permission, and I found a really helpful organisation called Parent Partnership where you can get advice on how to fight your way through the official jargon and which steps you have to follow to get your child statemented. Someone from the organisation will come to your house and help you to fill up the forms.

The letter about Matt was one of the hardest things I have ever had to do and it still haunts me. You have to write about your child from birth up to date and it seemed to put everything we had been through in black and white. Having to write down all the things that my son could not do for someone else to read really spelled it out for us. It seemed so condemning to be writing such a letter – the exact opposite of how you want to be as a mother. My protective side came out and I wanted to say 'but its ok I love him' as I couldn't bear other people to think badly of my child.

Once the letter has been written the education board has 12 weeks to give you an answer. The Parent Partnership representative will come to all the meetings in between and help you with form filling and with their help you don't feel so alone. I think they are fantastically helpful as I had to fight the school every step of the way and so I needed a lot of support. Once the decision has been made, which in my case was after a lot of hard work writing documents and going to meetings, the relief was amazing and I have to admit I felt smug when I thought about that head teacher. Little old me, who had had to learn from scratch, had won.

Tips for parents

- Get a copy of the Special Educational Needs Code of Practice from Department for Education & Skills (DfES) Publications **www.dfes.gov.uk** (0845 6022260).
- Ask to see local authority guidance/policy for special educational needs.
- Keep copies of all letters and take notes in meetings.
- Keep a diary of your child's progress and the difficulties you encounter.
- Go on a course – I found out about mine at the local library.
- Ask for help from Parent Partnership through your local education authority.
- Ring the education board and ask who is dealing with your case.
- Don't be afraid to speak out.
- Always ask if you don't know something or don't understand.
- Be really detailed in your letter to the education board.

- Find out your rights in the school. You are allowed to see the special needs policies of the school.
- Read the policies thoroughly and take notes if you need to.
- Don't think you are being a pain. You want what is right for your child.

Useful contacts

- **IPSEA** (Independent Panel for Special Education Advice) Organisation defending children's right to special education provision **www.ipsea.org.uk** (0800 0184016)
- **National Parent Partnership Network** – supports parents and carers of children with special educational needs. Contact through your local authority. They can put you in touch with an independent parental supporter, a trained volunteer who can help you through the statementing maze.

Benefits and how to get them

The complicated collection of benefits available and the range of eligibility for them can deter people from even applying, but you may well be entitled to more than you think, and it is only sensible to claim anything you are entitled to.

- Disability Living Allowance is a tax free benefit for people who need help with personal care and/or getting around. Find out more from the Department for Work and Pensions **www.dwp.gov.uk** Benefits enquiry line 0800 882200

- A guide to claiming DLA for children with brain disorders including ASD is available from **www.cerebra.org.uk**
- Disability Alliance **www.disabilityalliance.org** (020 7247 8776) for authoritative advice on benefits for disabled people.

Chapter 14

Treatments and therapies

There are lots of therapies and treatments around, some costly, some completely free. You never know what may work for your child: 'don't knock it until you have tried it' is my motto. Some things have worked for us, some have worked for other people, so what is included below can be seen as a collection of suggestions.

Massage

A daily massage has dramatically cut down on the incidence of tantrums for 12 year-old Alexander Lubbock, who is autistic, and his father is delighted that the treatment has made such a difference. 'A friend in our village who was aware of Alexander's constant anxiety offered to try to massage him every day for six months as an experiment, and it has led to an absolutely massive transformation. We are going to get her to go in and massage everyone at his school and try to monitor it fairly professionally to see if it works as well for everybody with this condition. It has been brilliant for Alexander; we went from about six tantrums a day to one a month. Initially we had sessions of 30 to 45 minutes a day and now he is down to three times a week, still with the same good effects. At first she came to the house and she had to follow him around and just rub his shoulders while he was at his computer and so on; pretty soon he was co-operating and now he goes to her house and just hops up on the massage table. It seems so logical that massage should be beneficial, I can't believe we never thought of it before. These children are always so tense and anxious and they have no reserves to deal with problems when they arise.'

Cranial osteopathy

Lesley Burton has found that cranial osteopathy has worked wonders for her son Eddie, who is four. 'I take Eddie for cranial osteopathy, which is absolutely marvellous. About four to five weeks after a session he just gets to the point where he is doing handstands all the time or bouncing everywhere and we realise it is time to go back to the osteopath and that demonstrably sorts him out a bit. We first tried it when he was about 18 months old and he didn't really like it, but there were noticeable benefits. I take him to the Osteopathic Centre for Children in Clerkenwell. Eddie was very difficult at first, he didn't like hands on his head or on his back and just wanted to leave, but we go regularly now and it is the making of him. You need to stick with these things if they are not too traumatic for them. With Eddie certainly there was a turning point when he suddenly seemed to realise that he always felt better after he had let them do the massage and now he will run in and let them get on with it. The Osteopathic Centre for Children is a charity where you pay what you can afford. They say that autistic children have got a very tight head and with

Eddie they say that the part of his brain that should deal with speech and language – the frontal lobe – is very tight and very restricted, which is typical of autistic children who are non-verbal. The treatment is so gentle and non-invasive, it has been a real success for us.'

The Osteopathic Centre for Children is at 15a Woodbridge Street, London EC1R 0ND, (0207 490 5510), and Phoenix Mill, Piercy Street, Manchester (0161 277 9911) **www.occ.uk.com**

Acupuncture

Long before her son Toby's diagnosis with Asperger's, Maddie Templar discovered how beneficial acupuncture could be for him. 'My acupuncturist suggested we try treating Toby when he was small, after I told her about his persistent cough and his behavioural problems. We found straight away that there were distinct benefits. It is fairly stressful being Toby, and he can't seem to get rid of the stress for himself, it just builds and builds until he has a tantrum: acupuncture really helps him. What seems to happen is that Toby's behaviour gets worse the day after his acupuncture, then somehow it clears and he can be relaxed for weeks until it is time to go for another session. He is very calm about the actual treatment, which is done while he watches television. For children up to about the age of ten (Toby is nine) the acupuncturist uses an electrical machine that passes a tiny current over the acupuncture points, so there are no needles for him to worry about.'

Find an acupuncturist through the British Acupuncture Council **www.acupuncture.org.uk** (0208-735 0400).

Speech Therapy

Speech therapy is invaluable for ASD children, but is not always easily available. If it is useful to your child and it is possible for you to do so, it is recommended that you should have speech and language therapy made as secure as possible on your child's statement as a special educational need in such a way that the LEA has a statutory obligation to provide it. The national shortage of speech therapists is highlighted by Lady Astor of Hever, whose autistic daughter, Olivia, has found speech therapy particularly effective. 'We couldn't get speech therapy through our LEA so I paid for a speech and language therapist for years. Olivia had weekly lessons, which were wonderful, and I learned a lot myself about how speech and language develop. Speech therapy and occupational therapy should be accessible to everyone, but there is a terrible shortage of therapists. It takes them so long to qualify and if they are paid on NHS rates they don't make any money at all so they all go privately. If the government doesn't give them a living salary, it is very difficult to get them to go and teach in schools. These services should be available for children who have any kind of special needs. They are the fundamentals – the building blocks – and they should be within education.'

Nutritional Therapy

A lot of ASD children have food phobias and some parents find it really helpful to get advice from a nutritionist. I have already talked about the problems I had getting Matt to eat anything new when he was younger. He is pretty good now, but I know that, for a lot of people with ASD, food remains a problem. The wilder reaches of the condition can be the home of eating habits that are, to say the least, erratic.

Parents who have battled with the nothing-yellow-ever diet, the exactly-the-same-thing-every-single-day-for-always diet, the only-white-food diet, the just-six-Smarties-and-nothing-else diet, and many more besides, will know how hard it is to ensure that basic nutrients get into the system, as nutritional therapist Sally Child is well aware. She recommends a full nutritional assessment if you have concerns, so that any testing, dietary changes and supplementation can be discussed and tailored to the individual child. As Sally says, 'there are several underlying factors which can affect the symptoms of an autistic child. I would investigate these and test accordingly. As they often eat very few foods and allergy/toxicity is common, increasing the range is important but difficult.

'I often have to start with blood sugar imbalances, which can cause cravings. Food intolerances will also lead to cravings and aversions to certain foods. Children become deficient due to the limited diet and poor absorption. They often have what we call a 'leaky gut', which aggravates neurotransmitter function and affects brain messages. In turn, the leaky gut is often caused by intestinal infections and deficiencies of friendly gut bacteria. Professor Paul Shattock at Sunderland Autism Research Centre has found that peptides for gluten and casein are often found in the urine of these children and indicate a toxic reaction to these foods. Many will improve when the foods are removed. This is of course not true of everyone and not all will respond; however, with proper supervision and the right replacement foods, improvements are seen and eye contact, affection and concentration seem to improve first. I would not recommend the removal of these foods without nutritional supervision. They are major food groups and it is important that the child is not deprived of foods unnecessarily. Other useful exclusions are sugar, yeast and additives and I nearly always advise this.

'It is virtually impossible to get them out of quirky fads as this is part of the condition and provides security, but it is possible to reduce them by balancing blood sugar levels. Asperger sufferers often only eat alone and at night, for instance. Protein is often low and fruit and veg non-existent. Long-term health problems from lack of fibre and anti-oxidants can be a real risk. Supplementation is very complicated and not recommended without supervision. Some remedies will be recommended as a result of test results. *Dietary Intervention in Autism* by Marylyn Le Bretton is a very good parental guide as to how to deal with the-day to-day problems of exclusion diets and weird eating habits. There is also info in my first book *An A-Z of Children's Health*: which has a section on autism. I would say that the older the child the less responsive they are to dietary intervention, but there is always something we can do to improve their nutritional status.' **www.nutritionfirst.co.uk** (023 8027 5646).

Music therapy

Music therapy is increasingly used as part of early intervention programmes for ASD children. It has been found that music can stimulate communication for them and music therapy is based on the idea that our innate responsiveness to music transcends handicap. Sessions will be either one to one or in a group and, as consistency is important for ASD children, will be held in the same place each week, in a quiet room with no distractions. Music therapy is not the same as music lessons – the child is not learning to play an instrument though they may acquire some musical skills during the sessions. The therapist uses percussion, tuned instruments or her own voice to respond in creative way to sounds produced by the child to make a musical 'language'.

Find a therapist in your area **www.apmt.org** (020-8440 4153)

www.nordoff-robbins.org.uk (020-7267 4496).

Sensory Integration Therapy

This method aims to help people whose senses are over-sensitive by flooding them with sensory experiences such as swinging, rolling, jumping and spinning. It is provided by specially trained occupational therapists. Further information from **www.sensoryintegration.org.uk** .

Auditory Integration Training

This is a complex, method which some people find very effective. It aims to help those with auditory processing difficulties by desensitising children to the sounds that bother them, leaving them more responsive to sounds in general, including speech. The treatment involves a number of sessions listening to music modified to avoid the individual hypersensitivities. **www.auditoryintegration.net**.

Relaxation

I have also heard of people who have had very positive results with relaxation classes – if you find one in your area, you could both go! If not, it might be worth investing in a relaxation tape and listening to it with your child. In fact, if your child likes to sit and listen, it might be worth considering meditation: I have heard of this producing surprisingly good results.

Some parents will want to leave the treatments alone, but, as Charlotte Moore, the mother of two autistic boys, writes in her fascinating book about them *George and Sam*, 'Powerlessness is bad for parents. If trying a diet or behaviour-modification programme makes them feel that their frustrated love for their child is being put to good use, then that's a good thing. I've tried a lot of treatments and have gained something from most of them.'

Chapter 15

Where to get help

Dealing with the Doctors

GP – Doctors can help a lot if you have a child with an ASD, but I feel that if they understood what we go through each day then they could help much better. They know the medical condition but not what it actually means to families like us. But if you are lucky enough to have a good GP who actually listens to you then half the battle is won.

- Do go to the GP and explain.
- See a doctor you know will listen even if it is not your usual doctor.
- Go back again if you are not happy with the outcome.
- Take in any observations you have done on your child's behaviour and habits if you think they might be relevant.

Consultant – You see the consultant a lot more than the GP, I found, and my consultant for Matt is fantastic and listens to all I have to say. I took the video of Matt's night terrors to him and he prescribed Melatonin. I was so relieved when it helped Matt out of the worst of his sleeping problems. You can also get help from them for school as they write letters and explain your child's problems.

- Don't be afraid of the consultants as they are there to help you.
- Tell them everything, even small details could help.
- Give them a video of your child if you cannot explain behaviour.
- Show them any written observations of your child you have made.
- If you are not happy with your consultant ask to see someone else.

Roles of the health professionals who might be involved with your ASD child

- **GP** – your first port of call for health services, will refer you on to specialists.
- **Health visitor** – specialist nurse with further training in child development, family health and welfare, will visit at home.
- **Community paediatrician** – doctor who is an expert in the health and development of children, especially those with disorders including ASD. Often diagnose ASD conditions and know when to refer child on to other specialists.
- **Paediatrician** – organises hospital services for sick children.
- **School nurse** – has expertise in conditions that may affect children's ability to learn; provides a link between school and health services.
- **Educational psychologist** – specialist who has studied how children learn and behave.

- **Dietician** – provides advice, information and teaching on nutrition and diets.

- **Portage worker** – uses a home teaching method originated in Portage, Wisconsin, has expertise in working with parents of pre-school children helping them with developmental difficulties; get information on the service from your health visitor.

- **Speech therapist** – can help promote the development of language and communication in people with developmental disabilities

- **Occupational therapist** (OT) – expert in understanding how ASD can affect day to day activities , gives practical advice to parents on how to reduce everyday problems faced by those with ASDs.

Useful-to-know abbreviations

This is a world awash with jargon. If you can't tell your PSAT from your SENCO you need to get to know your abbreviations ASAP.

- **S.E.N.** Special Educational Needs

- **S.E.N.C.O**. Special Educational Needs Co-ordinator

- **E.P.** Educational Psychologist

- **L.S.T.** Learning Support Team

- **A.E.O.** Area Education Officer

- **I.E.P.** Individual Education Plan – Teaching plan for children with special educational needs will set targets for your child to achieve within a given time and is regularly reviewed by the school

- **M.L.D.** Moderate Learning Difficulties
- **E.B.M**. Emotional &Behavioural Difficulties
- **E.W.O.** Educational Welfare Officer
- **P.S.A.T.** Pre-School Advisory Teacher
- **B.S.T.** Behaviour Support Team
- **L.E.A** Local Education Authority
- **C of P.** Code of Practice
- **V.O.** Voluntary Organisation
- **SP.L.D.** Specific Learning Difficulties
- **S.L.D.** Severe Learning Difficulties
- **P.M.L.D.** Profound and Multiple Learning Difficulties

Useful organisations

National Autistic Society, **www.autism.org.uk** (Helpline 0845 070 4004).

TEACCH: This programme aims to equip people with ASD to live and work more effectively at home and school, in the community and workplace. Various techniques and methods are used as part of individual plans specifically targeted at those with ASD and their families. The aim is to help them improve learning, social and language skills. TEACCH was developed in the US, details of the programme in this country from **www.autismuk.com**

OAASIS (Office for Advice, Assistance, Support and Informa-tion on Special Needs) for parents and professionals involved in special education.**www.oaasis.co.uk** (Helpline 09068 633201) has a number of very useful information sheets

Contact a Family: a national charity which supports families who have children with different disabilities and special needs. The organisation links with over 500 support and self-help groups, offering support and advice. Parents can be put in touch with a support group or another family whose child has a similar disability. **www.cafamily.org.uk** (Helpline 0808 8083555).

Chapter 16

What the future holds

There is only so much advice I can give on the teenage years. We are living through them ourselves at the moment, finding out as we go along. This is a bad enough time for all parents. ASD just adds a shed-load more complications. All I can do is tell you how we are coping – and really there are a lot more highs than lows these days – and hope it helps you.

Teenage life

It is bad enough for normal teenagers, with all those hormones flying around. Add those into the ASD mix and you can just imagine the problems and confusion that may ensue. Matt's early teenage life was, to say the least, eventful. He was invariably very easily led by others, which meant that some of his 'friends' egged him on and he got into all sorts of scrapes, for which he has had to be grounded from time to time.

- Now may be the time when you have to re-think some of the discipline you use. Do remember to reward good behaviour – ASD teenagers still need as much reinforcement as they did when they were younger.

- They may have a thirst for the new, but they still need the same reassurances and routines they have always had.

Trying new things and feeling safe by Matthew Keith Brealy

'I like to try everything as if you don't try it how do you know if you like it. I like to know what is going on all the time and when and how so I know what is coming next.'

Going out

Matt loves to go out with his brothers. Now Paul has a car Matt loves to go and meet Paul's friends and his girlfriend. I am very grateful for this as I think it will teach him a lot about socialising. Sometimes if Matt has been grounded for something (see above!) he will climb out of his window to go out. He loves the night sky and the thrill of being out late when he is not supposed to be.

- It is really important that ASD teenagers get good examples and practical experience of how to socialise, if that is what they want to do.
- Get a sibling to take him out socially so that he can see how to behave.
- Encourage your teenager to join a youth club, sports club or some other after-school activity.
- Some teenagers can get a lot out of half-term and holiday courses run locally – 'rock school', dancing, anything that interests them.

- You will probably take them out, too, but it is very important for them to get a taste of independent life without you if at all possible. If there are no siblings or dependable friends around, you could get a carer to take them out to the cinema, to a café and other places where they can see other people socialising.

Romance

Matt has not really had romantic feelings for girls, I think because he is a few years behind in some of his development. He always looked on girls as best mates, but I think he is starting to take more of an interest in them now. We worry about him being taken for a ride as he is very soft-hearted and would never see if he was being used. When he goes into town shopping with his own money he ends up buying all sorts of things for his friends and girlfriend. We would like to think that Matt could marry one day as we would hate for him to be on his own. But his wife would have to understand him and his condition. At the moment girlfriends are always on his terms, and that must be difficult for them.

- You and your partner can be a good example to a teenager embarking on relationships. Let him see you being considerate of each other's feelings, compromising with what the other wants and so on. Explain the give and take of a relationship to them. This is just as important as the facts of life.

Drink and drugs

We worry about all this, as Matt is not someone who would naturally say no. We had a drink and drug counsellor around to explain the topic to Matt and now he understands a bit more and tells his friends about the evil effects of drugs or how many units there are in a pint, but it would not stop him from drinking. I think in time, and with the good influence of his big brothers this will stop and I try not to worry too much.

If you have concerns in this area you can ask the special needs teacher to refer your child to counselling. This is for everyone but they will generally take account of special needs in what they do.

You can find information on drink and drugs on the internet or at the library and talk it through with your child.

Leaving school and thinking about the future

Matt is a pretty normal teenager in that he can't wait to leave school. He is going to go into building with his Dad. He likes it, and he could well be very good at it, so we hope that this will be his future. We are going to put Matt through a college apprenticeship in building. Building needs an understanding of shapes and structures and a love of order, ideally suited to some aspects of Matt's personality.

NVQ courses at college can be an excellent next step for some ASD children. They will be learning something practical and getting a trade, moving forward. For Matt the problem will be to keep him focused on a job. He will need short-term targets and a lot of supervision. We are lucky that we can help to push him towards a job that is tailor-made for his condition. Parents need to find the positives when looking for a job for an ASD person. For instance, many people with an ASD can concentrate on one thing for a very long time, so they can become very good at something they like doing.

- I would suggest that you look at NVQ courses as they are highly practical.
- Colleges will help with finding the right course. You could start with your special needs teacher, who should be able to put you in touch with the appropriate people at college.
- Of course, for the more academically gifted ASD children, university will beckon, as it does for most bright children. It is very important that you help your child as much as possible at this stage, with guidance from school or college, to find a sympathetic environment. They need to be comfortable with their choice, able to cope with their surroundings and to be protected from becoming isolated in their studies.

As ASD children get older you may find that it is hard to get the help you need – there is a real gap in provision for teenagers and beyond. We need courses to help parents battle through the teenage years. Once again this pinpoints how important it is to get the statement. Disability allowance can be so useful for young adults. Later our ASD children could be on their own and there is not enough support for them as so many respite-type places are shutting down. Once Matt gets to a certain age I know there is nothing more provided for him. He wants to experience life – we have to keep him safe. It is up to us to put in place what we can to safeguard his future.

When thinking about what the future may hold, bear in mind that your child may be able to claim the Disabled Students' Allowance (DSA). You can check the benefits situation at your local Jobcentre Plus office (Benefit Enquiry Line 0800 882200).

College and work experience

If they start a college course that will help provide a bridge into the outside world ASD teenagers are still going to need someone to fight their corner for them. 'I'm always completely upfront with work placement providers,' says Mary Thomason, who arranges work experience for students, many of whom have ASDs, at a centre for foundation studies in Cornwall, 'especially because students with even severe autism can look pretty normal. Potential employers have to be aware that there can be problems. For instance, students like this won't want people in their space, like things to run the way they should and can't cope easily with changes. One current student can't get to his placement on the bus because he says that if someone sat next to him who smelled really bad he just couldn't bear it. ASD senses can be so acute that things like that are really dreadful for them. The same boy, who is on work experience at a garden centre, can't cope with getting his hands dirty, so we have made sure that the employer understands that he needs to wear gloves all the time. You have to get placements that are sympathetic to their needs, and this is something that parents should bear in mind if they are not getting the back up from their child's college.'

Mary highlights the importance of getting your child's condition recognised while he is still at school. 'Children whose special needs are not recognised often fall through the net and can be really let down by the mainstream school system. Typically a child who finds things hard to grasp at school will find that teachers don't have time to explain and will probably end up mucking around in class and not get anywhere.'

This vicious circle is the problem with not getting diagnosed or statemented, and the many parents who go into denial about their child's condition are really not doing them any favours at all. 'They come to us with issues of communications skills and low self esteem. We do our best to build them up and from our foundation studies course we can refer them on to mainstream college and courses like plumbing or motor vehicles. The Sure Start programme can propel them in the direction of future employment with things like catering courses in a fully operational café where they can learn to take orders, operate the till, prepare food and wait on tables in a working environment.'

Useful organisations

- Your child can speak to a personal advisor at the local **Connexions** centre for advice on the next stage after school. This advice goes up to age 25 for people with learning difficulties. Connexions partnerships bring key youth support services together, so are a useful one-stop source of information and advice. **www.connexions-direct.com** (080 80013219)

- **Skill** is a national charity that provides opportunities for young people and adults with a disability in post-16 education, training or employment. **www.skill.org.uk** (0800 328 5050).

- **Foundation for People with Learning Disabilities** gives information on issues that affect learning-disabled people's lives, including education and employment **www.fpld.org.uk** (020-7803 1100)

The answer to a parent's question 'what can my child do next?' has to be that there is no real safety net out there to catch these young people when they get to the end of college. They need ongoing support when it comes to going out to work, and this is only patchily available around the country.

Children with ASD become adults with ASD, but their lives can be made much less challenging with appropriate education and support. While there are some things that will never be easy for Matt, there is not necessarily any limit on what he could do.

Bringing up Matt has certainly been a roller coaster ride for us, but that means lots of ups as well as downs. We are very proud of ourselves to have survived the ride. The roller coaster will never stop for us but as a strong family unit we know the future will get better for us all. As a family we are very proud to see Matt grow into a happy, outgoing, loveable teenager with a difference! We will never stop guiding him through his life and I am sure Matt will never stop teaching us!

The Future by Matthew Keith Brealy

'I am going to be a builder I am going to be a bricklayer. But I do not know what I will be doing in the future that is the whole thing about the word future.'

We hope you have found this book useful – we have enjoyed writing it.

Email Jackie and Bev: **enquiries@whiteladderpress.com** with any feedback.

Useful Contacts

Please note You can also find this list on our website at www.whiteladderpress.com.

National Autistic Society, **www.autism.org.uk** Helpline 0845 070 4004.

Early intervention

CHAT test details can be found on the National Autistic Society website www.autism.org.uk or the PEACH (Parents for the early intervention of autism in children) website **www.peach.org.uk**.

The Elizabeth Newson Centre in Nottingham for specialist diagnostic early assessment (01623 490879) **www.sutherlandhouse.org.uk**.

PECS further information from Pyramid Educational Consultants UK Ltd, Pavilion House, 6/7 Old Steine, Brighton BN1 1EJ (01273 609555) **www.pecs.org.uk**

PEACH (Parents for the early intervention of Autism in Children), The Brackens, London Road, Ascot, Berkshire SL5 8BE (01344 882248 **www.peach.org.uk**)

Early Bird Centre, 3 Victoria Crescent West, Barnsley, S. Yorks S75 2AE (01226 779218 details on **www.autism.org.uk**

Home-Start **www.home-start.org.uk**.

National Portage Association **www.portage.org.uk**

Hanen **www.hanen.org**

Makaton **www.makaton.org** (01276 61390).

SenseToys **www.sensetoys.com** (0845 2570849)

Education

Contact a Family Helpline 0808 808 3555 **www.cafamily.org.uk**.

Education Otherwise.**www.education-otherwise.org** (helpline 0870-7300074).

www.he-special.org.uk has resources for home educating a child with special educational needs

Network 81 – working towards inclusive education for children with special needs – helpline 0870 770 3306

Parents for Inclusion **www.parentsforinclusion.org** helpline 0800 652 3145

Advisory Centre for Education (ACE) **www.ace-ed.org.uk** (helpline 0808 8005793)

Bullying Online **www.bullying.co.uk**

Statementing and Benefits

Department for Education & Skills (DfES) Publications **www.dfes.gov.uk** (0845 6022260).

IPSEA (Independent panel for special education advice) Organisation defending children's right to special education provision **www.ipsea.org.uk** (0800 0184016)

National Parent Partnership Network –supports parents and carers of children with special educational needs. Contact through your local authority.

Disability Living Allowance :Department for Work and Pensions **www.dwp.gov.uk** Benefits enquiry line 0800 882200

A guide to claiming DLA for children with brain disorders including ASD is available from **www.cerebra.org.uk**

Disability Alliance **www.disabilityalliance.org** (020 7247 8776)

Therapies

The Osteopathic Centre for Children, 15a Woodbridge Street, London EC1R 0ND, (0207 490 5510), and Phoenix Mill, Piercy Street, Manchester (0161 277 9911) **www.occ.uk.com**

The British Acupuncture Council **www.acupuncture.org.uk** (0208 735 0400).

Sally Child, Nutritrional Therapist, 127 Ashdown Road, Chandlers Ford, Eastleigh Hampshire SO53 5QH (023 8027 5646) **www.nutritionfirst.co.uk**

Association of Professional Music Therapists (UK), 61 Church Hill Road, East Barnet, Herts, EN4 8SY; (020 8440 4153): www.apmt.org. The Nordoff-Robbins Music Therapy Centre, 2 Lissenden Gardens, London, NW5 1PQ; (020 7267 4496: **www.nordoff-robbins.org.uk**

Sensory Integration Therapy **www.sensoryintegration.org.uk** .

Auditory Integration Training **www.auditoryintegration.net**.

Help for teenagers

TEACCH: details of the programme in this country from www. autismuk.com

OAASIS (Office for Advice, Assistance, Support and Information on Special Needs) for parents and professionals involved in special **education.www. oaasis.co.uk** Helpline 09068 633201

Connexions partnerships bring key youth support services together, so are a useful one-stop source of information and advice. **www.connexions-direct.com** (080 80013219).

Skill is a national charity that provides opportunities for young people and adults with a disability in post-16 education, training or employment. **www.skill.org.uk** (0800 328 5050).

Foundation for People with Learning Disabilities gives information on issues that affect learning-disabled people's lives, including education and employment **www.fpld.org.uk** (020-7803 1100)

Faces for the fridge

You can cut out or copy these faces and turn them into fridge magnets. When your child is too emotional to express their feelings in words, they can point to the face that indicates the way they feel, just as Jackie does with Matt (see page 21).

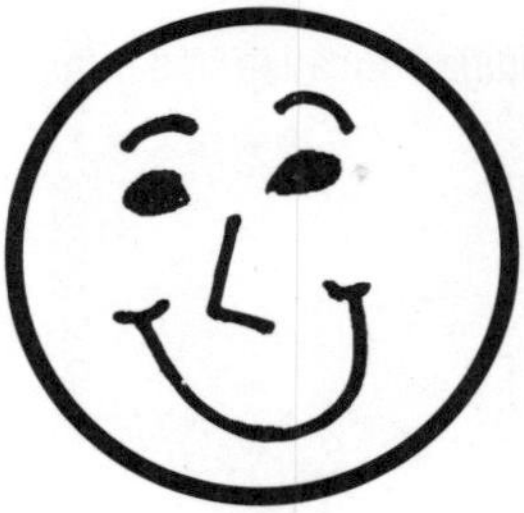

Happy

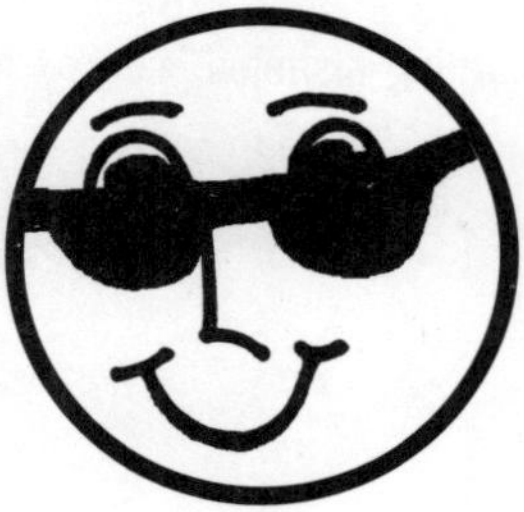

Cool

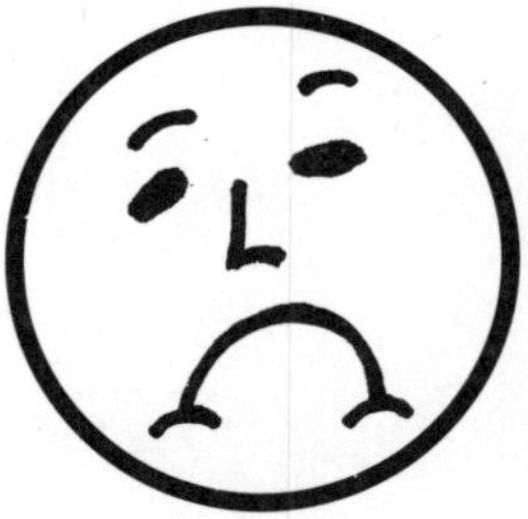

Sad

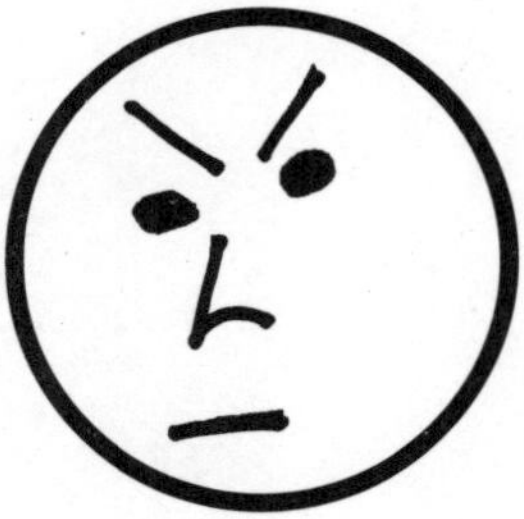

Angry

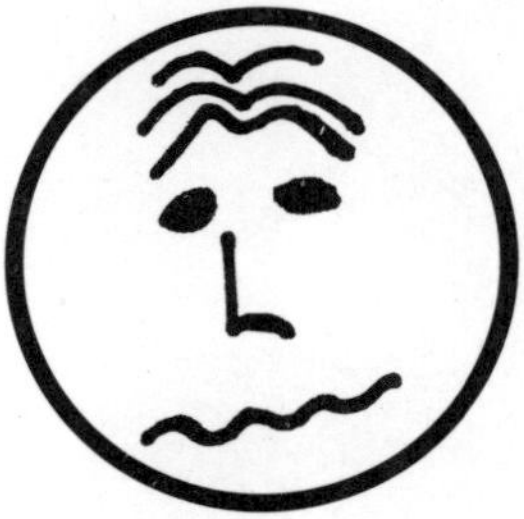

Worried

Index